The Dimension of the Present Moment

Miroslav Holub was born in 1923 in Plzeň, western Bohemia, the only child of a lawyer and a high-school teacher of French and German. He attended a gymnasium specializing in Latin and Greek, so that Homer and Virgil were the first poets he read carefully. He was brought up to admire Goethe and Romain Rolland and French poetry in general. After graduation in 1942, he was a labourer at the Plzeň railway station. When the war was over, he studied science and medicine at Charles University, Prague, and worked in the department of philosophy and the history of science, and also in a psychiatric ward. He became an MD in 1953 and thereafter specialized in pathology. In his student years, he started to write poetry and became an editor of the scientific magazine, *Vesmír*, the equivalent of *New Scientist*. In 1954, he joined the immunological section of the Biological Institute of the Czechoslovakian Academy of Science and obtained his PhD the same year his first book of poems appeared. He became associated with the literary group Poetry of Everyday. A prolific writer, he produced almost one book a year until 1969. He was widely translated – fortunately, since between 1970 and 1980 he became a non-person and his work was available only in translation. He worked as an immunologist in New York from 1965 to 1967 and in Freiburg in 1968. He has published over 140 scientific papers and three monographs – the last, *Immunology of Nude Mice*, in 1989, in the United States. He has written fourteen books of poetry and five collections of essays and other prose.

The Dimension
of the Present Moment

Essays by MIROSLAV HOLUB

Edited by David Young

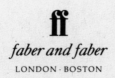

faber and faber
LONDON · BOSTON

First published in English in 1990
by Faber and Faber Limited
3 Queen Square London WC1N 3AU

Photoset by Wilmaset Birkenhead Wirral
Printed in Great Britain by
Richard Clay Ltd Bungay Suffolk

'The Dimension of the Present Moment' and 'Poetry and
Science' were first published in FIELD, Contemporary Poetry
and Poetics, Oberlin College Press, Oberlin, Ohio.

'Shedding Life' was first published in *Science 86*.

'The Dog that Wanted to Return' was first published in
Sagittal Section, FIELD Translation Series 3 (1980).

Miroslav Holub is hereby identified as author of this work in
accordance with Section 77 of the Copyright, Designs and
Patents Act 1988.

A CIP record for this book is
available from the British Library

ISBN 0-571-14338-5

Fais ce que tu peux – la plupart ne le fait pas!

Uncle Gottfried in Romain Rolland's *Jean Christophe*

Contents

Preface

Like the contemporary science Miroslav Holub clarifies, celebrates and uses to enhance the range and depth of his poetry, this collection of his essays in English translation is the product of teamwork and collaboration. Though I have acted as general editor and as co-translator of many of these essays, often working, as I do when translating Holub's poems, with Dana Hábová and with the author himself, a number of other translators – Rebekah Bloyd, Steven Culberson, Patricia Debney, Stuart Friebert, Jarmila and Ian Milner, Maria Ondrasova, Vera Orac and Ewald Osers – have had a hand in one or more of these essays, so it seems best to supply a list:

'The Dimension of the Present Moment' – Hábová/Young
'Pre-human Humanity' – Milners/Young
'Shedding Life' – Hábová/Debney/Young
'A Path into Darkness' – Ondrasova/Young
'Man and Animals' – Ondrasova/Young
'Tissue Culture' – Milners/Young
'From the Intimate Life of Nude Mice' – Hábová/Young
'The Dog that Wanted to Return' – Hábová/Friebert
'Perhaps They'd Better' – Hábová/Young
'Giving Us Heart' – Hábová/Young
'The Emperor Inside Out' – Osers/Young
'The Statue' – Hábová/Young
'Pedestrians and Cells' – Hábová/Young

'A Walk in the Forest' – Hábová/Young
'Men with Knives' – Hábová/Young
'The World in Miniature' – Orac/Culberson/Young
'Visible Microbes' – Hábová/Young
'Growing Up' – Bloyd/Young
'Transplantation' – Hábová/Young
'If Kant' – Hábová/Young
'On Kindness' – Orac/Culberson/Young
'Maxwell's Demon' – Hábová/Young
'Windmills' – Hábová/Young
'Poetry and Science' – Friebert/Young

This list, however, does not reflect the substantial role Holub himself has played in guiding, encouraging and correcting his translators. There is scarcely an item to which his name should not be silently added (since he refuses more formal recognition). Also missing is the name of Georgia Newman, my wife. Her knowledge of current science, and her eye for improvements and clarifications in these texts, have proved invaluable and timely. Putting these essays into their more or less final form – some were still being revised and expanded at the very last minute in November 1989 – I have tried to make Holub's remarkable prose clear and succinct without losing any of its idiosyncratic qualities. Successful or problematic, the process has been exhilarating, and I am grateful for the opportunity it has presented.

David Young

The Dimension of the Present Moment

The fact that I cannot imagine the present moment has always worried me. By the present moment I mean a conscious individual state or process, an experience; the larger-scale present is rather easier to grasp. What is a moment, what is this moment in which I evidently exist, unlike nature, which according to Whitehead's famous quotation does not exist in a moment?

As a matter of fact, I can imagine eternity much better, particularly when looking up at the sky or the ceiling of a waiting room.

For me, the present moment has always been a dimension without a dimension; it bothered me so much that I once wrote an essay and entered it in a students' union literary competition. I came in fifth, but only theoretically, because immediately after the announcement of the awards the students' union was sort of annulled, and my inner concept of the present moment was thus further impaired.

I have finally found satisfaction in recent data of experimental psychology. The present moment lasts three seconds. In our consciousness, the present moment lasts about three seconds, with small individual differences.

The basic experiment is very simple: the tested subject is presented with a brief light or sound signal; the person is asked to reproduce the signal. If the signal lasts less than two seconds, the reproduction is always slightly longer. If the signal lasts almost three seconds – or a little over two seconds in some persons – there is a sudden reversal and the tested person interprets the signal almost accurately. If the signal takes more than three seconds, the tested subject shows a tendency to shorten the repeated version. Five-second signals are often reproduced as three-second ones and mistakes increase with the duration of the signal.

This shows that stimuli lasting more than three seconds cannot be maintained by our consciousness as a whole; we are somehow compelled to correct them. Therefore, the subjective present can be defined and it is as characteristic and real as the size of shoes you wear.

The so-called metronome test produces the same results. The metronome, the ruthless commanding officer of our musical attempts, ticks away, as we know, at any set interval, and each stroke is the same. However, listening to a metronome, we can easily make ourselves perceive one stroke as stronger, the following one as weaker. The alternation of subjectively stronger and weaker strokes produces the time-joined formation 'tick-tock, tick-tock'; two subsequent strokes form a unit of perception – they become inseparable, they belong together to such an extent that if one tick or tock suddenly disappeared, we would hear it in our mind. And, again, this is true only if the time interval between the two strokes does not exceed two or three seconds. When it does, we are no longer capable of forming subjective accents and patterns.

Naturally, the discovered dimension of the psychological present moment could have considerable practical consequences. For instance, in the arts it would be like a universal key. Every musical composition, especially of classic or romantic tradition, has its basic tempo, which the musician either keeps or breaks. This tempo should be in some relation to the dimension of the present moment. Musicologists acquainted with the above-mentioned psychological findings have so far examined Mozart's music. Several independently run tests have demonstrated that Mozart's musical motifs average two to three seconds.

Research in the lofty province of traditional poetry has also shown what is called the 'present-time frame'. In 73 per cent of all German poems, from Gryphius to Hugo von Hofmannsthal, lines read aloud last from two to three seconds. Lines lasting over four seconds are, or can be, divided into shorter segments, and the reader makes a slight but noticeable pause in the middle of the line. Analysis of interpretations of Goethe's poems shows that a line having fewer syllables is read markedly more slowly, or with a longer pause. Greek and Latin epic hexameters are divided by a strong caesura into two three-second segments and the same time unit has been found in different English, French, Japanese and Chinese metred poetry (F. Turner and E. Pöppel, *Poetry*, August 1983).

The three-second poetic LINE of Turner and Pöppel appears to be a 'carrier-wave' of traditional poetries in any language system; poetry as an art of language is presumably processed by the left brain lobe. But the metre based on the LINE carries meaning in the fashion of a picture or melody and integrates the right-brain processing into the left-brain activity. Thus 'the metered language comes to us in a "stereo" mode, simultaneously calling on the verbal resources of the left and the rhythmic potential of the right' brain hemispheres. In addition, metre 'clearly synchronizes the speaker with the audience and provokes a "rhythmic community" essential to the "social solidarity" ' – the great presence and simultaneity of people – which is about the best that poetry can do. The authors make in their magnificent essay a strong case for the 'cultural universal' of metred poetry as opposed to 'free verse'.

I have undertaken some micro-research on the Czech TV programme *The Sunday Night Poems*. The poems were by Nezval and were well recited; a line lasted almost exactly three seconds, shorter lines were prolonged by slower reading or pauses, longer ones were reduced by a quicker tempo. I was almost frightened and felt I ought to apologize at the Poet's Corner, but what for, really? The famous poet had simply stuck, intuitively, to the given ancient law which he applied to his free verse. I may be wrong – as usual – but I can't escape the feeling that at least in some linguistic and cultural contexts the LINE concept applies to free verse too. In some free-verse systems the LINE may be subdivided into meaningful sub-structures, but basically a good free verse operates with the three-second 'experience parcels' which are enforced by 'intellectual breathing pauses', resemblances and echoes in single units.

Besides, free verse in our cultural context operates within a strong metred poetry tradition and is perceived against the background of traditional poetry patterns not as a negation, but as a variation of the ancient 'poetry habit'. Contrary to Turner's and Pöppel's conclusion about the social role of free verse, in our experience free verse has emerged as a tool of broad social concern in poetry, as a carrier of political accents stripped of the mellowing and mollifying effect of traditional metres; it is an instrument of intellectual analysis centred on meanings, 'experience parcels' of general meanings, rather than on private feelings: I do not know any bureaucratic establishment which would prefer (as Turner and Pöppel suggest) free verse. I know of many which just love the traditional rhymed verses, because they do not say so much and rest in the traditional private domain of agreeable songs.

And here we get to common everyday speech, in which experts (Pöppel's school in Munich) have found involuntary insertions of roughly millisecond pauses which may be prolonged in some cases up to tenths of seconds that break up the verbal flow every three seconds. They say that during this 'intellectual breathing pause' the following speech unit is being pre-programmed, in lucky individuals even a thought might be pre-programmed. That goes for children as well, unless they are threatened by parental or school pressures and censures. And the same goes for Chinese speakers, because the subjective present moment is independent of language, grammar and syntax. Those who read their speech from paper for accuracy are an exception. The segmentation of speech by intellectual breathing pauses is so fundamental that it is almost impossible to imitate. The unpleasant character of a memorized statement simulating human speech consists in the very fact that it lacks time units, structure and natural pauses.

The dimension of the psychological present probably does not concern only speech; speech is a phenomenon suitable for demonstration and measuring. I dare to think that present-time frames are implied even in the process of thinking and feeling, and everything that is contained in the consciousness takes place in those tiny facets, in switching on and off, fading in and out, emerging and submerging. You cannot get into somebody's head, you might just as well ask a meal worm how to bake bread, but I can at least ask if, when you are thinking, your thinking is an uninterrupted, uniform flow. Is it not rather a procession of brief tests, pauses, criticisms of the preceding thoughts, new trials?

And: how long are we happy? Using my well-tested and reproducible model of taking off tight shoes, I cannot say I was happy for ten minutes after taking them off. Maybe those few seconds, followed by a reflection in the way of – oh, great, and also, damn, those shoes are tight! And another couple of seconds . . .

I strongly suspect that we simply happen in segments and intervals, we are composed of frames flickering like frames of a film strip in a projector, emerging and collapsing into snake-like loops on the floor, called the just-elapsed past.

And since we live permanently convinced that the past is past and it will be amended, and the future, even the immediate future, will certainly be even better and with fewer errors, since we live permanently removed from and critical of our own past, permanently removed from and in the hope of our oncoming future, the present-time frame of several seconds is the only unconditional manifestation of our ego.

In this sense, our ego lasts three seconds. Everything else is either hope or an embarrassing incident. Usually both.

...man Humanity

...was subjected to a small act of physical
...ng in line to buy a book of Robert Lowell's
...d it hard to imagine a situation from which
...s' would be wholly absent. If a priest were to
...wafers while serving communion, I suppose
...that those who had already received it might
...f aggression from those who hadn't. Even
...s, for that matter, especially the Greek gods,
...precarious. Getting your face slapped wouldn't
...nake a myth: Kronos, who ate five of his children
...throne, was cast into eternal darkness by Zeus
...le ten-year struggle. Later on, Zeus exterminated
...vice, the first time because they were ridiculously
...cond, following Prometheus's innovation, because
...dangerously powerful. Myths were made, we're
...r image; the gods didn't behave differently from the
...and cultured Athenians, who wiped out the entire
...n of the island of Melos during the Peloponnesian
...e civilized public, familiar with myth and history, likes
...bout aggressive human nature; it's satisfying because
...can help their 'nature', just as they can't help being
unable to make vitamin C from sugar residues.

But, you can ask, exactly what kind of nature *do* human
beings have when man in his sapient form is about 300,000
years old, while human civilizations, as we know them today,

have existed only for about one-tenth of that time? During that brief moment in the history of nature the hereditary equipment of this long-lived mammal couldn't have changed that much. Darwinian natural selection wasn't working substantial changes on us: brain mass, rationality and intelligence haven't changed, according to the geneticist Susumu Ohno (1978). The inborn intelligence of the individual shouldn't be confused with what we owe to cultural and social evolution: what looks like individual intelligence is really the collective intelligence of the species. Culture is an attribute that is passed on in a speedy, Lamarckian way. Konrad Lorenz demonstrates this fact through the example of language: the neurosensory apparatus for human speech was produced by an evolution of the species dating back to pre-human forms, but its full operation requires the existence of a culturally developed language, one that we spend our lengthy childhood acquiring. In that sense man as a species has no 'human nature', only a history, or, as Arthur Gehlen one said, man is by nature a cultured creature.

If man, in the present sense of the term, is 300,000 years old, his biological essence goes back several million years – about five, in fact. According to the molecular clock, we're separated by that much evolutionary time from the chimpanzee and the gorilla; in the sequence of amino acids in proteins we differ from these primates by 0.8 per cent, according to King and Wilson.

Thus it is that our biological essence comes from the very depths of nature. It's not our fault if we're aggressive; it's those hominids inside us, with which we're often in conflict.

Ohno agrees with the cultured public that our 'inner conflicts, brought about by numerous contradictory demands made by individual genes in the human genome, constitute the most important asset of man', and that 'inner conflicts . . .

were the driving force that set *Homo sapiens* upon the unique path of social evolution' and 'are responsible for the formulation of the whole noble concept of "soul" by man'.

Among the genomic contradictions, Ohno includes teeth that were suitable for forest apes feeding on fruits and berries but that were found unchanged among pre-human populations hunting wild animals in savannahs and eating omnivorously. He also cites the survival of mutally aggressive behaviour, characteristic of male animals living in a harem structure, among hunters who require mutual co-operation for survival. 'The combative urges of human males, induced by our post-pubertal androgen activation of a specific set of genes', are the basis, for him, of both historic and prehistoric killing. Thus a lion who acquires a lioness and promptly kills her cubs from the previous litter is not really different from Shakespeare's Richard III, murdering his brother's sons, or Edward the Black Prince, who exterminated all the inhabitants of the conquered city of Limoges.

What makes this picture even grislier is the fact that the hypothetical ancestor had a 'carnivore's mentality' without being a beast of prey. As Lorenz demonstrates, a professional carnivore would have built-in inhibitions against any excess killing and eating of his own species, unlike the omnivorous creature, basically non-predatory and harmless, that can even be driven to cannibalism.

As for the nature of evil, the growth of the brain may be partly to blame. Arthur Koestler believed that the bestiality that surfaces in acts of murder and war is a result of the accelerated growth of the human brain, which has enlarged so rapidly in the last two million years that the cerebral cortex, the seat of reason, loses its control of the emotive, animal centres in the deeper layers. Influenced by the views of the

1920s, Koestler considered the brain to be both the instrument and the cause of the great leap forward in humanization.

Dart's scenario, formulated in the 1920s and based on the discovery of two-million-year-old Australopithecines, held that these small creatures, erect and walking on two legs, abandoned their woodland herbivorous habits, created weapons from bones and stones, weapons their hands were now free to carry and that could aid their insufficient teeth, and then, to meet the increased demands on their intelligence required by hunting, expanded their brains. Their skulls bore traces of suspicious violence. From killing baboons it was a small step to the killing of their brothers of the same species, as Kubrick's *2001: A Space Odyssey* nicely demonstrates.

Our direct ancestor might thus be this murderous post-ape; no wonder our history drips with blood. Our biological essence is that of Cain.

But is it really?

In the early 1970s it was shown that the Australopithecine evidence, the crushed skulls and pierced holes, was the work of leopards and collapsing cave ceilings. Louis Leakey, who discovered most of the hominid skeletal remains, turned up no traces of murder. In Kenya, Glynn Isaacs found two-million-year-old campsites – home bases, to be more precise – to which the hominids returned repeatedly, bringing with them food, including dead animals (whose bones bear the traces of stone knives). In these places they made their knives, as splinters demonstrate, and peacefully kicked the bucket. In other words, these little two-legged guys, non-apes, non-humans, shared their food among themselves, so that 'sprained ankles and fevers ceased to be fatal diseases' (S. L. Washburn). Because weapons that could be used to hunt larger game appeared only a million years ago, and because waddling on two legs was an inefficient way to overtake prey, and because a lion or a leopard could easily be frightened by making noises or waving thorny branches, these hominids probably didn't hunt. Instead they gathered fruit and appropriated animal carcasses killed by beasts of prey. Their smallish brains weren't up to much more than that anyway. They started walking erect so they could drag home their goods, not so they could kill.

For appropriate development and selection (genes mutate, individuals are selected, a species develops, according to David Hull's summary of orthodox Darwinism) they had a good two million years before them. In 1974 Don Johanson discovered in Ethiopia the more than 3.7-million-year-old skeletal remains of Australopithecines, first the little girl 'Lucy' and then whole families, forms that, long before Dart's hominids, walked on two legs and carried their completely ape-like heads erect. Then in 1982, in the same area, Desmond Clark found the remains of a boy who was about sixteen. They were 400,000 years older. There were also the traces of a fireplace. A similar creature left sets of footprints on a stone plateau found by Mary Leakey in 1976. A family of three was running through mud, fleeing from an erupting volcano. The ashes preserved the footprints. This creature lived on fruits and meat, as the traces found on the teeth of Johanson's hominids by an electron microscope indicate. And their hands could delicately grasp things and drag loads, but couldn't firmly clutch a weapon.

The greatest advance in humanization, then, was walking on two legs and sharing food, apparently accompanied by a change in sexual behaviour. According to Owen Lovejoy (1981), the reason why a sturdy male returned home must have had to do with a monogamous union with a single female who — in sharp contrast to the rutting of apes — was continuously attractive and sexually receptive. This enabled the species to reproduce more often and in greater number, since the females didn't have to stray too far from the home base and could take care of a larger number of dependent offspring. Behaviour relating to increased reproduction is a trait that develops and stabilizes itself very rapidly. The union of pairs constituted a decisive advantage in development over the apes, and it probably led to the beginning of individualized facial features and emphasized sexual characteristics, among which we may at least mention Aphrodite's breasts ... According to Tanner, these Aphrodites preferred peace-loving and co-operative males who were prepared to bring food home and protect the family. Thus the inherited tendency to co-operation gained a developmental advantage over tendencies to masculine conflict and competition.

More than two and a half million years after Johanson's hominid, the brain's weight was doubled. And that was in the African human branch, *Homo habilis–Homo erectus*.

Now we have an alternative scenario for the biological essence of humanization. No murderous post-ape, no King Kong brandishing his just-invented heavy weapon, but a tame and rather unsophisticated creature who drags home the shopping, looks after the wife and kids, protects the weak from banishment and unnecessary death, uses his voice not only for shouting signals to co-ordinate the hunt but for essential household communication, and is selected for his ability to co-operate, not for his aggressiveness. Lorenz rightly foresaw that human qualities could develop only in friendly groups. Only in such conditions was there room for the creating of artefacts, from small knives to wall pictures, and for that most human quality, humour. Cains never laugh. And because 'ritualized behavior only reproduces in tribal development the given modes of social behavior', we started to behave like human beings for the reason that four million years ago those little two-legged, four-foot-tall after-apes began to act that way. Our biological essence is pre-human humanity, not aggression. The wear and tear of later history is a deviation from the norm, not the biological norm itself.

But tell that to the Zeuses, Richard IIIs and the like. I didn't even venture to say it in the line waiting for poetry.

Shedding Life

A muskrat, also called musquash, or technically, *Ondatra zibethica zibethica* Linn. 1766 — the creature didn't give a hoot about nomenclature — fell into our swimming pool, which was empty except for a puddle of winter water. It huddled in a corner, wild frightened eyes, golden-brown fur, hairless muddied tail. Before I could find instruments suitable for catching and removing muskrats, a passing neighbour (unfamiliar with rodents *per se*, or even with rodents living in Czechoslovakia since 1905), deciding he'd come across a giant rat as bloodthirsty as a tiger and as full of infections as a plague hospital, ran home, got his shotgun, and fired at the muskrat until all that was left was a shapeless soggy ball of fur with webbed hind feet and bared teeth. There was blood all over the sides and bottom of the pool, all over the ball of fur, and the puddle of water was a little red sea. The hunting episode was over, and I was left to cope with the consequences. Humankind can generally be divided into hunters and people who cope with consequences.

I buried the deceased intruder under the spruces in the backyard, and, armed with a bundle of rags, I went to clean up the shooting gallery. The swimming pool doesn't have a drain, so the operation looked more like an exercise in rag technology, chasing the blood north, south, east, west, up and down. Chasing blood around an empty swimming pool is as inspirational as listening to a record of Haydn's 'Farewell Symphony' with the needle stuck in the same groove. I became very intimate with the blood in that hour, and I began to daydream about it. The blood wasn't just that unpleasant stuff that under proper and normal conditions belonged inside the muskrat. It was the muskrat's secret life forced out. This puddle of red sea was, in fact, a vestige of an ancient Silurian sea. It was kept as an inner environment when life came ashore. Kept so that even – though it's changed to a radically different concentration of ions, a different osmotic pressure, and different salts – the old metabolism hasn't needed too much reshuffling.

In any case, the muskrat was cast ashore from its own little red sea. Billions of red blood cells were coagulating and disintegrating, their haemoglobin molecules puzzled as to how and where to pass their four molecules of oxygen.

The blood corpuscles were caught in tender, massive nets of fibres formed from fibrinogen, stimulated by thrombin that was formed from prothrombin. A long sequence of events occurred one after the other in the presence of calcium ions, phospholipids from blood platelets, and thromboplastin, through which the shot arteries were trying to show that the bleeding should be stopped because it was bad for the muskrat (though in the long run it didn't matter). And in the serum around the blood cells, the muskrat's inner-life signals were probably still flickering, dimming and fading out: instructions from the pituitary gland to the liver and adrenals, from the thyroid gland to all kinds of cells, from the adrenal glands to sugars and salts, from the pancreas to the liver and fat tissues – the dying debate of an organism whose trillions of cells co-exist thanks to unified information.

And, especially because of the final chase, the adrenalin and the stress hormone corticotrophin were still sounding their alarms. Alarms were rushing to the liver to mobilize sugar reserves, alarms were sounding to distend the coronary and skeletal muscle arteries, to increase heart activity, to dilate bronchioles, to contract skin arteries and make the hair stand up, to dilate the pupils. And all that militant inner tumult was abandoned by what should obey it. Then there were endorphins, which lessen the pain and anxiety of a warrior's final struggle, and substances to sharpen the memory, because the struggle for life should be remembered well.

So there was this muskrattish courage, an elemental bravery transcending life.

But mainly, among the denaturing proteins and the disintegrating peptide chains, the white blood cells lived, really lived, as anyone knows who has ever peeked into a microscope, or anyone knows who remembers how live tissue cells were grown from a sausage in a Cambridge laboratory (the sausage having certainly gone through a longer funereal procedure than blood that is still flowing). There were these shipwrecked white blood cells in the cooling ocean, millions and billions of them on the concrete, on the rags, in the wrung-out murkiness. Bewildered by the unusual temperature and salt concentration, lacking unified signals and gentle ripples of the vascular endothelium, they were nevertheless alive and searching for whatever they were destined to search for. The T lymphocytes were using their receptors to distinguish the muskrat's self-markers from non-self bodies. The B lymphocytes were using their antibody molecules to pick up everything the muskrat had learned about the outer world in the course of its evolution. Plasma cells were dropping antibodies in various places. Phagocytic cells were creeping like amoebas on the bottom of the pool, releasing their digestive granules in an attempt to devour its infinite surface. And here and there a blast cell divided, creating two new, last cells.

In spite of the escalating losses, these huge home-defence battalions were still protecting the muskrat from the sand, cement, lime, cotton and grass; they recognized, reacted, signalled, immobilized, died to the last unknown soldier in the last battle beneath the banner of an identity already buried under the spruces.

Multicellular life is complicated, as is multicellular death. What is known as the death of an individual and defined as the stoppage of the heart – or, more accurately, as the loss of brain functions – is not, however, the death of the system that guards and assures its individuality. Because of this system's cells – phagocytes and lymphocytes – the muskrat was still, in a sense, running around the pool in search of itself.

Not to mention the possibility that a captured lymphocyte, when exposed to certain viruses or chemicals, readily fuses with a cell of even another species, forgetting about its previous self but retaining in its hybrid state both self and non-self information; it can last more or less for ever there, provided the tissue culture is technically sound.

Not to mention the theoretical possibility that the nucleus of any live cell could be inserted into an ovum cell of the same species whose nucleus has been removed, and after implantation into the surrogate mother's uterus, the egg cell will produce new offspring with the genetic make-up of the inserted nucleus.

The shed blood shows that there is not one death, but a whole stream of little deaths of varying degrees and significances. The dark act of the end is a special and prolonged as the dark act of the beginning, when one male and one female cell start the flow of divisions and differentiations of cells and tissues, the activation of some hereditary information and the repression of some other, the billions of cellular origins, endings, arrivals and departures.

So in a way the great observer William Harvey was at least a little right when he called blood the main element of the four basic Greek elements of the world and body. In 1651 he wrote: 'We conclude that blood lives of itself and that it depends in no ways upon any parts of the body. Blood is the cause not only of life in general, but also of longer or shorter life, of sleep and waking, of genius, aptitude and strength. It is the first to live and the last to die.'

Blood will have its way, I thought, wringing out another rag.

It is the colour of blood that makes death so horrible. People and other creatures (unless they happen to be the likes of a shark, hyena or wolf) have a fear of shed blood for this reason. It is a fear that hinders further violence when mere immobility, spiritlessness and breathlessness can't. A fear that keeps the published photographs of a killing or slaughter from being true to life. The human reaction to the colour of blood is a faithful counterpart to the microscopic reality, the lethal cascade we so decently provoke by the final shot in the right place. There are an extraordinary number of last things in anyone's bloodbath. Including a muskrat's. And if any tiny bit of soul can be found there, there is not one tiny bit of salvation.

They say you can't see into blood. But I think you can, if only through that instinctive fear.

Lucky for the Keres, the goddesses of bloodshed, that no one concerns himself with the microscopy of battlefields; lucky for the living that molecular farewell symphonies can't be heard; lucky for hunters that they don't have to clean up the mess.

A Path into Darkness

'Men fear death, as children fear to go into the dark,' wrote Francis Bacon in his essay 'Of Death' (1612), 'and as that natural fear in children is increased with tales, so is the other. Certainly, the contemplation of death, as the wages of sin and passage to another world, is holy and religious; but the fear of it, as a tribute due unto nature, is weak.'

In the European tradition of thinking, nature is somehow associated with life, birth and being, as suggested by the term 'natural' itself. Staying in nature has the emotional connotation of being a living thing among living things, something not contradicted even by observation of the sexton beetle as it opposes nothingness by turning the end into a beginning. In traditional thinking, death is perceived as an opposite and a negation of life, as a metaphysical illness entailing physical illness. This has had its repercussions in the not-too-intensive search by the natural sciences for the causes of death which, as a rule, end in hypotheses that variously blame metabolic errors, disappearance of a special type of inherited feature, nucleic acid degeneration, and the accumulation of harmful substances.

The somewhat poetic identification of death with the phenomenon of a cadaver gave rise to the textbook dictum regarding the immortality of unicellular organisms that leave no cadaver when dividing into two, more or less equal, daughter cells. However, regarding death as an end to the existence of an individual, it makes no difference whether a cadaver or two paramecia or two anthrax bacilli are left; the parent cell has in any case ceased to exist; there is no more of her and there will be no more of her. It's just that it's a little less tragic, since the end of one is the beginning of two. And the entire process warrants plasticity and variability of the species, since the unlimited existence of an individual would lead also to unlimited permanence of the basic properties of its own body, a condition that would prove destructive in the variable conditions of being in this world.

In the biology of multicellular organisms, which concerns us a little bit more, death is inherent in several respects. First, all cells capable of division end their individual existence on the birth of two new cells. Second, purposeful and strict integration of cells into tissues and organs requires, beginning with the earliest stages of development, predetermined or programmed destruction of some cellular unions. Degradation of cells during embryonic life is a prerequisite for morphological and functional maturation. If the cells between our fingers had not died out, we would have no fingers but a hand like a pan. If the cells of our embryonic adrenal glands had not perished, we would have no functional adrenals in adulthood. If some cells with embryonic functions did not pass away, they would give rise to tumours compromising the whole body.

Third, as has been demonstrated over the past twenty years, the whole body, the whole biological unit of the multicellular, strictly integrated body, is endowed with a programme of death, perhaps even with a programme of death-timing, which can of course be modified but not outwitted. For many reasons, it is probably not expedient – expedient from the point of view of survival and adaptive potential of the species, that is expedient from the point of view of nature herself – for us to hang around here once we have fulfilled our main genetic assignment, that is the creation of daughter organisms.

This point is best illustrated in the octopus: the female octopus, whose sexual life embraces other remarkable features that enliven popular science books, lays eggs, thus activating certain secretions from an area of a photosensory gland. The secretion is deadly, killing the octopus. If the respective gland is removed, as demonstrated by Wodinski, the octopus lives on. Thus she has an organ of death right inside herself, and if this is not pleasant for the octopus in question, it is probably pleasant for the octopus as a species.

This phenomenon apparently has nothing to do with decent mammals, including the law-abiding readers. Perhaps only apparently. There is, in fact, such an organ in us too. An organ starting to vanish upon our reaching sexual maturity, despite any preventive and therapeutic measures. The organ is the thymus, an organ virtually unmapped in terms of its import-ance and, consequently, somewhat unpopular. Unfortunately, this organ is the centre of the body's immune system, with cells that pass through it enabling infallible recognitions of self and non-self. Absence of the thymus makes identification of viruses and malignant cells less possible, less accurate. The gradual degradation of the thymus and its cells therefore constitutes a programmed opening of the body to the invading marches of death, regardless of which illness death chooses as its route. While it would be theoretically possible to supply properly instructed thymic cells to each individual, it is unfeasible because of transplant immunity, that is incompatibility of tissues and cells, and because of the factor referred to as Hayflick's cellular clock: in 1961 Hayflick and Moorhead published the results of experiments suggesting that all cells of the body are programmed for a number of divisions that cannot be exceeded. As a result, all cells of the body are encoded, and this is true even under conditions of tissue culture (that is, without regulation from the body as a whole) encoded with a programme of self-destruction. This encoding applies to thymic cells as well, in which case the consequences of Hayflick's clock are perhaps even more illustrative than elsewhere, although the limited number of cellular divisions anywhere in the body makes its death a generally multifactored process.

'If there were no death, life would have to come to an end,' summed up Professor Charvat, speaking to Haskovcova in 1975. Therefore, if nature contributes something to our philosophy of life today, it contributes the obverse of death – the death of an individual as a precondition of the life of other individuals, tragic death as a precondition of biological optimism. Considering death as a source of philosophy and inspiration, it perhaps would be useful if we tried to work from a somewhat better understanding of nature and the natural essence of things, an inspiration better than that aroused by a walk in a park in autumn, or by listening to funeral ceremonies, or even 'education against death', that is instruction about the psychological, ethical and metaphysical aspects of death, an experiment that, in a test by Baulis and Kennedy in the United States, succeeded in reducing normal high-school students with fifty years of life expectancy to abject panic. The point is that while we are the only animal with an awareness of death, the main defence we have is relative obliviousness. And I don't think one should or could do anything to this individual 'ignorance'. In a way, it is an approximation of biological or genetic supraconsciousness, in which the question of individual death is not central. After all, each individual inspiration is steered by control centres of emotion in the hypothalamus and limbic system that have evolved in the unimaginable process of natural selection and are its result and record.

From the point of view of volume of information, then, both the hypothalamus and the limbic system, as well as the thymus, are wiser than the mind of a philospher, a fact one may find embarrassing but also somewhat reassuring.

And if Wallace Stevens said that 'death is the mother of beauty', it may not be entirely inevitable to take that in the sense of autumnal morbidity and cemetery secrets – which are easier to deal with in poetry than in vigorous youth. It may also be understood in the sense of biological optimism.

Man and Animals

The basic moral principle – of man's responsibility for someone or something within his control – is regularly raised in discussions about the protection of the environment and the preservation of endangered species of animals and plants. Made absolute, the same principle demands that everything we found on the planet, in the process of growing wiser, should be preserved on the planet. Had we been wise already in the Mesozoic period, we would have had to do our best to preserve the archaeopteryx and the dinosaur. Yes, and the giant horsetails and lycopods as well. Also the Eohippus, so we wouldn't have invented the harness. Oh yes, also the Australopithecines, so we wouldn't have perhaps evolved . . . Well, we had other problems at that time.

Unfortunately, one cannot observe the above principle strictly: as the Dutch biologist and author Dick Hillenius quipped, if we are sorry for the elephant and the tiger, why aren't we sorry for the tapeworm, the typhoid bacteria, the rats and mice?

Moral considerations and emotional responses tend to stop working somehow as soon as one's own interests are at stake. Are we less responsible for annoying and harmful (with 'harmfulness' often being a rather relative notion) insects than for storks and tits? Seen from this point of view, the uproar caused by pesticides was a little hypocritical. N. E. Borlaug, the Nobel Peace Prize laureate and the 'father of the Green

Revolution', stood up very vehemently against 'hysterical environmentalists' who predicted a doomsday through poisoning by chemical agents, and defended their use because the living standards of millions of people depend on it. By the way, he noted, out of the 1,100,000 animal and 350,000 plant species, civilization-related activities endanger only several dozens (for example, nine species of reptiles and amphibians in North America); as regards hundreds of thousands of species, we do not even know whether they are endangered by us, by 'nature' alone, or by nothing at all. If pesticides caused the death of 100,000 head of game each year, this would trigger off massive campaigns. However, the same number is killed on US roads and motorways annually and very few people care to protest since the environmentalists must also travel somehow . . .

There's no question that one cannot condone unnecessary and, for practical reasons inexcusable, interventions into life on the planet, or relentless and indiscriminate entrepreneurial nihilism. On the other hand, it is impossible to regard, for example, the animal inventory of the planet as a museum collection in which all exhibits must necessarily be on display. We are responsible for the planet as a whole and as a viable system. Viability in planetary dimensions assumes civilization's activities, which have never ushered in such sweeping changes as those that triggered the Jurassic calamities of large reptiles.

It follows from this that moral considerations must incorporate practical aspects, perhaps with a sigh, but, still . . .

Our moral and emotional relations to animals are symbolically reflected in the situation of experimental animals. To put it euphemistically, the experimental animal is a bit like a sacrifice to the Powers of Human Progress; the first experimental animal, in this sense, was Abraham's scapegoat, sacrificed for the well-being of mankind.

While common sense admits the need for animal experimentation and takes for granted the benefits of, for example, medical advances enabled by experimentation, it singles out, on the other hand, the process of experiment *per se*, called vivisection, as suspicious. Tender-hearted souls see an experimenter as a somewhat unscrupulous and stigmatized individual. This is true even though domestic animals in any farm or countryside household usually get much harsher treatment. I have never noted that geese are anaesthetized or that rabbits are killed by injection instead of by techniques originally employed by Neanderthal man. Here again, the attitude taken by the public to animal experiments contains a touch of hypocrisy: while absolutely insisting on painlessness or the indivisibility of being alive, the public is reluctant to concede the limits of this demand in everyday practice.

This situation is reflected in a special manner in the life stories of Charles Bell and François Magendie. Bell was a Scottish surgeon and anatomist who was at Waterloo. On seeing the consequences of cerebral injuries on battle victims, he was among the first to realize and describe the association of certain parts of the brain with certain parts of the body. He discovered the difference between afferent and efferent neural pathways, the former carrying sensory impulses to the brain, and the latter commands for movement from the brain. His observations should have been verified by experiments on living animals; these, however, Bell never dared to perform. In 1822, he wrote in a letter:

I should write a third communication on nerves, but I cannot get any further without performing some experiments that are so unpleasant I am afraid of performing them. You may well consider me foolish but I cannot convince myself completely I am authorized by my character or by my religion to do these crucial things — and what for? — for anything but a little bit of egotism or self-glorification . . .

Bell did not use the argument of human interest and progress. His moral position was thus unshakable and may serve as a model of humanism much better than Waterloo. However, his historical role was fulfilled only thanks to his — say — moral antipodes, who 'convinced themselves completely . . .'

His antipode was François Magendie (1783–1855), conducting experiments without too many scruples. He would simply cut, or dissect, his contemporaries claim, with apparent pleasure and indisputable virtuosity. From the point of view of Bell and other tender-hearted souls who, as a rule, do not become war-time military surgeons, he was a complete villain and a sadist. Magendie is said to have demonstrated repeatedly on a rabbit, from which he would excise, bit by bit, cerebral tissue, observing how this gradually limits perception of pain and how paralysis proceeds. He was very proud of mastering these procedures even though the rabbit, not anaesthetized (logically, since Magendie could not demonstrate anything under anaesthesia), tossed about, at least at the beginning. Magendie even argued against anaesthesia generally, citing such fabricated or superstitious assertions as, for instance, that ether may induce untoward hallucination or unexpected sexual urges, posing a risk to the performing surgeon.

None the less, Magendie verified Bell's observation and hypotheses: on trassecting animals' afferent nerves, the muscular response disappeared. This gave rise to the Bell–Magendie law, one of the foundation stones of theoretical and practical medicine in today's meaning of the word. An idealist and a sadist were combined by history into a single concept. At the same time, the sadist became a hand moved by the idealist's ideas. As Péguy remarks, idealists will have clean hands if they have hands at all. It is appropriate to add that, while Magendie acknowledged Bell's precedence, Bell regarded Magendie as a thief of his ideas.

From an ethical point of view, the only possible solution to the problem of an experimental animal is also an analogy to the merger of Bell and Magendie. Bell's attitude is no doubt a priority. Only on condition that there's no alternative to tackling a key problem (which qualification cannot be the result of consideration by an individual, but must be a matter of general consensus by the professional and peer public) is it possible to proceed to inflict pain, minimal pain, within the shortest time possible. And this with awareness that it is still pain and that only a triumph over more intense pain, over the pain of many people, will justify the sufferings of several experimental animals.

Both in the issue of the preservation of animal species and in the issue of sacrifice and pain in a biological experiment, our considerations are eventually guided by the interest and advance of mankind. Application of the criteria of humanity and the use of the term 'humanity' itself are based on a fundamental difference, even an opposition, between man and the rest of existence. However, the definitions of 'interest' and 'benefits', as well as that of 'humanity', are somewhat intricate.

Various evolutionary levels of human society, various historical stages of man, perceive advance and humanity from quite different perspectives. Even the same person may qualify 'human' and 'humane' behaviour in a different manner, according to the situation. Virgil's pastoral eclogues would have run a little differently had he been recruited as a legionary taking part in the last Gallic genocide. Generally speaking, the attitude to slaughterhouse animals is in most cases still more humane than that of the Roman and Punic cohorts massacring each other in the dust of Carthage.

Application of humane criteria alone and in single situations is shaded and diversified by a hierarchy of objects. A layman, as well as a biologist, is firmly and *a priori* convinced that there exists a progression of organic forms, as anticipated even by Aristotle, and that there exist species more valuable and less valuable for man, just as there exist species biologically and psychically closer to and more distant from man. Therefore, as Konrad Lorenz retorted, the mounting of moral protest to the killing of a living thing is arranged in a very confused order, from cabbage to fly to frog to dolphin to cat to dog to chimpanzee: 'The genesis of a higher form of life from a simpler, preceding stage implies for us an increasing value, a fact as indisputable as our own being.' Most importantly, I should say, the response of a chimpanzee to any infliction of pain is much more understandable, more 'humanlike', than that of a newt, even though it may hurt both of them equally.

This hierarchy also governs the criteria of animal protection, even though the preservation of an expedient and biologically harmonic environment may, in some situations, depend more on the unicellulars than on the elephants.

Finally, separation of human interest and the human criterion from the rest of nature presupposes human morality as a completely new quality, even though its predetermination by a network of instincts has recently become, thanks to the investigations of Lorenz and his disciples, obvious.

The moral code that man observes or wants to observe or

should observe in relation to animals (just as in his relations to others of his kind, to people) is not as unique as one might be tempted to think, judging by ancient beliefs. The biological basis (in other words, functionality or expedience) of the inhibition of aggressiveness among animals, and the basis of the human taboo or even of rational morality, are apparently very similar. Konrad Lorenz gives examples of the inhibition of aggressiveness: the male wolf under no circumstances attacks or bites a female wolf. Nor does a male lizard. Adult individuals of the overwhelming majority of vertebrates never attack, not only their own offspring but also the offspring from other colonies of the same species. Offspring and females are taboo, untouchable — the only difference being that the inhibition of aggression is transmitted and inherited among animals as an instinct, while it is transmitted by cultural tradition in man.

The cultural transmission of taboos, rules and inhibition of aggression carries exclusively human features: while transmission by heredity and the acquisition of new qualities (which can be as well referred to as information) through mutation and natural selection is relatively very steady, the human mode of transmitting information is extremely effective and rapid. It took the primitive four-toed horse Eohippus, Waddington maintains, sixty million years to evolve into the horse. By comparison, the technical development of automobile and aircraft spanned thirty-odd years. The changes in aggressiveness and inhibitions in the behaviour of an animal species take place within a geological time scale. New features of the human moral code of man emerge or disappear, thanks to the means of information, thanks to language and its derivatives such as the press, radio and television, virtually instantly.

Human responsibility for the living things in this world is

not due to a spark of enlightenment in an 'ethical animal': it is due to the extent, plasticity and speed of information, knowledge and judgement based on the same species-defined expedience and species-determined awareness of progress that guide the slow and lagging steps of behaviour and action in animal species.

We are, one might put it, from the same mould. The only difference is that we know it better and more distinctly than the others. Hence our responsibility, not only for mankind, but also for animal kinds.

Tissue Culture or, About the Last Cell

At a not-so-small celebration of some small research successes, an investigator engaged in the cultivation of tissues in glass exclaimed, '*In vitro veritas*!' Although his exclamation was produced not by the kind of media used in tissue cultivation (designated by such unpalatable abbreviations as RPMI and MEM), but by a medium toxic to tissue cultures though very conducive to celebrations, the saying stuck in my mind. How much truth can one find 'in glass'? After two billion years of unicellular existence, life set out on the road of cellular specialization, of division of labour and functions among cells, and the unification of cells into larger and larger and more and more self-regulating organisms. What can be revealed by having cells and cellular unions thrown back into a bowl filled with some ingenious, yet always somewhat deficient, proto-sea?

Malevolent, malignant cells in a tissue culture tend both to grow indefinitely and at the same time to baffle the investigator, once they can no longer do any harm to their original carriers. It's just good manners in oncologic or virologic research to try to establish continuous, permanent lines from them. Some comply, but many seek revenge by giving rise to mysterious phenomena caused by the reciprocal contamination of cultures. The most notorious cells of this kind are those of one Henrietta Laks, which have been growing *in vitro* as HeLa cells since 1951 and displaying a downright cosmic eagerness and offensiveness; helped by some less than vigilant and diligent technicians they have managed to sneak into as many as ninety other tumour cell lines all over the planet. HeLa profit from the lack in tissue cultures of one of the few constraints that pertain in biology, namely that a mouse is a mouse, a monkey a monkey, and only Henrietta Laks is really Henrietta Laks. That's why HeLa cells have run up millions of dollars in damage in American and German, Soviet and Chinese laboratories. Not to mention the moral harm caused by the many people who have lied, deliberately or inadvertently, about the very nature of their HeLa-contaminated cultures. In such ways, malevolent cells really can undermine the truth *in vitro*.

Normal, non-malignant cells are so reluctant to grow in cultures for any length of time that they are rather unlikely to be mixed up, even by the most ingenious technicians; they don't wait that long. In their allotted time *in vitro* they may reveal some of the truth about themselves. Certainly, in a suitably formed culture, cells designed to ingest will continue for a time to ingest, cardiac-muscle cells will pulsate rhythmically for a while, cells capable of division will divide some more, and nerve cells will emit the refined and delicate projections along which impulses are carried. Cells designed to synthesize antibodies can be made to synthesize antibodies, especially after fusing with tumour cells, thereby forming almost immortal cell lines from a single cell and thus creating one of the most productive instruments of modern biology, the monoclonal, absolutely pure antibodies. The cells in refined large cultures produce interferon or promote the production of viruses for vaccines.

The cells of tissue cultures tell us much that is true about themselves, then, and fulfil their defined functions. But they know roughly as much about the music of the organism as a bunch of crocuses knows about Mendelssohn's 'Spring Song' and vice versa. Perhaps, apart from the cells of connective tissues, which provide intricate networks at will, the cells in the glass suffer not only from lack of nourishment but from lack of information. They will try to achieve natural contacts, search for one another, issue signals and combine into primitive tissues. But they will lack their primary meaning, which induced the origins of multicellular bodies. They'll be worse off than an ant without its ant-heap, or a man all alone in a sound-proofed, blacked-out room.

Observing tissue cultures by microscope is immensely satisfying because it is one of the few means of direct insight into the modes of cellular life. At the same time it's rather sad and disturbing: you are witness to the ultimate deprivation of units of life. Just a little bit less oxygen, only a fraction more acidity, an error in just one amino acid – and there's nothing but a vast, silent cemetery, an almost bare battlefield after a battle in which all sides lost.

And in this witnessing there is one very general truth, one very basic truth with two faces, which can be seen in the glass by means of the microscope.

Anyone who cultivates tissues knows that the first hours after sowing or planting the cells in the medium are the worst. The most primitive factors, like the very nature of the water (bringing with it many technical problems of distillation and elimination of ions) or, similarly, the nature of the embryonic serum which is usually needed (carrying with it many of the life problems of the donor calf) can be the origin of the culture's undoing. Even with the best water and the least toxic serum, the first hours see a great hecatomb among the cells, a vast selection of the individuals who will endure and those who won't, the latter being the majority. In tissue culture, cells don't live 'in general', but are selected by a process that can be foreseen and controlled only with difficulty. The life of cell collectives in the culture is always sub-total, never total. The relative immortality we achieve in our cells involves only a narrow selection of cells, of whatever kind. Only tumorous cells show a general growth – with appropriate care, an unlimited growth – as a living memorial to the long-dead donor, sometimes with his or her initials, as in the previously mentioned HeLa cells. Normal cells grow for only a limited time, set by the programmed number of possible cellular divisions. And, finally, even the culture of the selected, fittest individuals – obedient to the basic law of life – perishes. That is one side of the above-mentioned truth.

The other side is that even in what can be designated as a dead culture one can always find some isolated little cellular thing capable of life and self-preservation. After the most awful trials of freezing and thawing there is always, still smouldering somewhere, a little cellular life – one cell in a thousand, one in a million, in ten million, but it's there, waiting for some kind of salvation. While life in cell culture is far from complete, death at any given moment is never 100 per cent effective either.

A memorable exception to this rule was the experience of one research worker in a laboratory I visited some years ago. She repeatedly cultivated lymphocytes that within a day were completely and uniformly dead. She had it in for them, called them malevolent cells, but she never reported her strange, deathly talent, and subsequently departed for practical life. No one ever succeeded in repeating this experience. After any kind of mistake there always remains a fragment that is not worth preserving but that illustrates the other side of the truth:

collective death is almost always sub-total, not total. There's always some individual who gets out of hand – maybe it hides, maybe it's forgetful, maybe it's especially capable, or especially incapable.

When we throw out waste tissue culture, we may be sure there's always something very small in there calling for help. It's no longer the voice of the tissue culture, the simplified vocal register of life, but rather the whisper of the last, lonely, useless, but none the less hopeful hope. No longer really science but still poetry. No longer what is law-carrying, but rather something beyond it, a statistically meaningless and negligible exception.

The incongruous whisper of the last living cell: if you have time, don't discard it; go to the microscope and look at the orphan cellular movement in the dish, and listen. You won't hear anything that's essential for the ear of biology, but after a while you'll recognize that it is a cosmic sound; that in spite of all the sadness of the single deserted and condemned cell, there is in its mere occurrence something optimistic for cells in general. Always, there is somebody who trangresses death. And even though it would take the Dead Water (which, according to Erben's tale, joins together the remnants of dismembered corpses) and the Live Water (which gives new life to reconstituted crows and crown princes) to make a tissue culture from the abandoned cell, or a mouse from the tissue culture, in the fact of the last cell, the essence emerges – an essence which assisted the onset of cellular life billions of years ago.

The statistically insignificant exception is in most experimental situations unimportant for science. But it is rather important for man. It is that *in vitro veritas*, even though nobody hears it, usually – because, usually, there is no time to listen.

From the Intimate Life of Nude Mice

We used to have a colleague who was hard-working but peculiar. After everybody had gone home and the laboratories were empty, he would take a few cages with mice from the institute's animal facilities, put the males together with the females and watch the goings-on. He also used the institute's official stationery to write to the United Nations Secretary General and to the Pope, demanding the preservation of world peace. These petitions did not help his popularity in higher places, as the higher places believed peace had to be preserved, as it were, from up there downwards, not vice versa, and after some time we lost our colleague. We lost a colleague, the mice an appreciative observer.

For us, his penchant for observation, let us say, sexual dreaming, was nothing but a peculiar diversion, not sought out by the busy person, who has enough worries and activities as it is. It was not until years later that we came across a problem with which our former colleague could have helped to some extent. That is, unless he kept on writing petitions at the same time.

The problem was to find the zero time. That is the zero time in mice, meaning the moment – well, perhaps not the very moment, but at least the hour – of conception. The whole development of the embryo occurs at a rather impractical speed. For twenty-four hours the egg, an egg among other fertilized eggs, is in the state of one cell; in two days there are four to sixteen cells, the egg travels through the Fallopian tube, and it is only after four to five days that it settles in the uterus and begins to grow like mad, so that between the fifth and tenth days the lump of stem cells differentiates into the overall building plan of the embryo and its organs. It is a bit like a lump of iron ore turning into a space shuttle. In fact it is the profoundest wonder we can still imagine and accept, and at the same time it is so usual that we have to force ourselves to wonder about the wondrousness of this wonder.

When it is ten days old, it is a complete plan of a mouse, and in another nine days it *is* a mouse, sitting pretty like a little pink worm in the nest, together with six to seven siblings, and mother mouse sits on top, doing her best to produce good mouse milk.

It makes sense that if you want to capture the first aortic arch, you need an embryo exactly eight days old, and if you want to capture the first buds of legs–hands, it has to be after exactly nine and a half days, and if you want to see how masses of cells move to the diminutive rudiment of the thymus, it has to be exactly between the eleventh and eleven-and-a-halfth days.

Eleven-and-a-halfth day since when?

It is, in fact, a wicked but poetic licence of nature to make this basic step of determining a new individual so indeterminable. You can wash out the fertilized eggs from the Fallopian tube and implant them in a culture like microscopic pancakes; you can fertilize eggs *in vitro*; you can mix two embryos to make a chimera; you can transfer eggs and early embryos into the uteri of prepared foster mothers (pseudopregnant recipient does not sound any better); and you can even transfer a cloned gene, by a microshot of DNA into the primitive nuclei of the fertilized eggs, or with the aid of viral carriers, and produce a transgenic mouse, a mouse carrying new genetic information determined by man. All this can be done without long experimental discussions with mother nature and parental lines of mice, but none of this can be used to get normal mice with a normal intra-uterine development and to get a sufficient number of such mice, baby mice or embryos.

For that we need mouse sex, but it is difficult to interfere even in fellow human beings' sex lives, let alone in those of such distant creatures.

The secret of getting close to the moment of mouse impregnation without peeping is by means of a time estimate based on probability and statistics. And the rules of probability and statistics are of course often broken, even by disciplined individuals, where sex is concerned.

The whole trick of co-ordinating mouse sex is to keep the mice in a permanent cycle of light and darkness, and to take into account that the female ovulates once every four to five days, three to five hours after it gets dark, let us say when night sets in. The males then behave in their notorious way (and let us presume that in mice these matters are less complicated by spirituality and other neuroses common in people), and with increased diligence, roughly in the middle of the night, that is during the dark period of a night lasting ten hours, which means one to two hours following the ovulation of a female selected according to the external signs of the oestrus – a determination about as accurate as trying to guess fever from pink cheeks. The female who had some fun is identified in the morning by the so-called vaginal plug, which is about as accurate as the measurement by Ancient Roman mothers of the neck circumference of their daughters after they had been on a Roman date: and that itself is not a total superstition, because a biggish endocrine upheaval occurs when sex takes place, and it makes itself felt on the thyroid gland.

The result? Some 50 per cent of the mouse females are in the family way, a result we cannot describe as a great victory of human spirit over the mouse. I would rather say it is the victory of mouse sex over cold statistics.

But let us imagine now that the target of our efforts is a ten-day embryo of the nude mouse, so-called nu/nu, a really hairless mouse without a thymus, and on top of that variously affected in its endocrine activities. Affected to such an extent that some ten years ago a nude mouse with offspring from a nude husband was a rarity. Today this happens even in our improved conditions, which are not very favourable either for nude mice or for naked apes (Desmond Morris's term).

Unlike people, nakedness in mice is not particularly arousing sexually, so this female mutant, this mouse mutant nude, is not especially attractive for mouse males. In these matters, everything is governed by smell, and the only minute advantage of the nude mouse is that the female is almost never identical with the male in some tissue antigens, and mouse males, perhaps even the nude ones, prefer this dissimilar mouse female, smelling the dissimilarity from the urine.

The behaviour of nude mice in the prescribed cycle of light and darkness, and in the prescribed setting, is even less predictable than the behaviour of ordinary mice, and some 50 per cent of gestations are a very academic dream. Their behaviour also varies because they are always cold whenever the temperature drops below 30 to 32°C, because they are less aggressive in most situations, and because many are latently sick from viruses and protozoa, so to expect that they are going to do the expected is to ask too much from fate.

You can manufacture a chimeric mouse, something between a nude and a hairy mouse, by merging early embryos, but you cannot very well produce normal nude baby mice of a required age. If there is mouse poetic licence in this, there is also a small piece of freedom and justice, since the mice, which are practically the work of human hands and human organization, have their privacy, their intimate life and their uniqueness, and we cannot meddle in these things.

Even if our colleague spent three to five hours sitting and watching the nude mice after the beginning of the dark period, when he would not see much anyway, and even if he were trained to distinguish the success or failure of the act in question, he would be of little help.

So, not expecting any graces from nature, we must expect that basic grace from the poor nude mouse.

The Dog that Wanted to Return

Destinies of experimental dogs are not obvious until the moment they're delivered to the site of the experiments. They arrive in a closed station wagon, filled with dog-dread and mystery formulated by philosophers in such questions as, Where do I come from? Where am I going? Canines formulate these questions by leaving puddles and whining.

At the experiment site, the dogs are enclosed in cages according to their races and natures. The dog-keeper, assisted by a hose, is the sun of their days; he serves the indefinite dog stew, their sole suitable recreation. The rest consists of howling, attempts to jump three metres high, pass through the wire netting sparrows can penetrate, mate with dogs of the same sex, murder dogs of smaller size, and defend their cages by barking hysterically. For such is the natural disposition of a dog. Even the cages have to be watched over, natural dispositon dictates.

A dog is selected for experiments if for two weeks he has manifested a healthy condition, and if his weight is satisfactory. He is then taken on a leash by the keeper. The joy in his tail is immense, and all co-dogs envy him with all their hearts. The dog on the leash thinks it's time for his walk with his master again. This walk, however, is very long. It is never terminated and therefore never repeated.

Once, though, a small spotted dog with a white chest and a bell collar slipped out. He ran away. He was fleeing. For such is the natural disposition: to flee a place of fear, of whining and desperation.

He was running in ever-increasing circles around the cages. The circles were irregular, depending on how he was chased. He was chased by the keeper. He was chased by fences. He was chased by buildings. He was chased by trees and bushes. He was chased by the grass and flowers. He kept running and he realized he feared fences and buildings and trees and flowers. And while fleeing and fearing, he discovered he even feared his keeper, although the man had been the sun of his days. And that is why he didn't let anybody catch him. And that is why he stopped being an experimental dog and became a dog. A dog-as-such.

Such is the natural disposition of things: having lost predetermination, we lose our attributes.

The small spotted dog-as-such crawled through the fence, and set out into the streets. Yet there was not one house, car or stone he recognized. He met the local dogs accompanied by their masters. He did not recognize them either. Yes sir, I'm from far away, from the Moravian border, he said to himself, trying to explain it, if a dog-as-such can say anything at all. He didn't recognize, he didn't belong, didn't belong to the streets, dogs, days or nights. Such a dog is dog that does not belong.

Not from hunger, but from not-belonging this dog realized he had to go back. He abandoned the windy breezes of the streets and corners, he crawled through the fence, he recognized trees that had chased him, he felt the scent of dog-fright and predetermination, he heard the hysterical barking of those who had guarded their cages from the invasion from Aldebaran, he recognized the station wagon and the stew bucket, and not seeing any keeper he approached the cages, welcomed by the raging hatred of co-dogs. He was quiet, for a dog without an attribute has neither a voice of advice nor a voice of warning. He crept towards his cage and tried to get in, he tried to pass through the wire netting penetrated by sparrows. He tried with his right paw and with his left. He tried to dig, he tried to jump three metres high. He tried it from all sides and he tried in vain. Such is the natural disposition of things: it's impossible to re-enter one's destiny.

So he spent the night under old rabbit hutches, in the closest proximity to his cage, lay down and rolled into a ball-as-such.

In the morning, he avoided the keeper. At dusk, he returned to his cage. His flight became a circular pilgrimage from the non-existence of freedom to the indubitable existence of the cage. For such is the natural disposition of things: even though it's impossible to go back, it's imperative to keep going back.

Moreover, belonging is contained in a dog's mind, while being-as-such is not contained in it.

This dog belongs to this cage and this fear.

Nights, when villainous cats lurk behind the bushes, and the aggressive stomping of rabbits can be heard, the eyes of the small dog under the rabbit hutch radiate the red, reflected light of lamps and planets, and the canine supernatural life: endlessly, until on his circular pilgrimage an unknown car hits him, and he becomes an experimental dog angel, an angel which will receive a leash and be weighed and selected for the experiment on the subject of the Influence of Eternity on the Natural Disposition of a Dog.

Perhaps They'd Better

Tumours arising from nerve cells appear at a very early age; these cells are differentiated during embryonic development, and do not divide after birth. Tumours originate from the remains of the persisting embryonic nerve tissue. A case in point is retinoblastoma, the tumour arising from the retina. Retinoblastoma affects one out of 18,000 children. It can spread from the optical nerve to the brain, and kill.

Twenty years ago retinoblastoma had a virtually fatal outcome. Since then surgical and therapeutic techniques have advanced, so the affected eye, or eyes, can be removed, along with a section of the optical nerve, to prevent the movement of malignant cells into the brain. According to the statistics of the American Cancer Society, 85 per cent of these children survive more than five years, which in the language of the science of tumours equals recovery. That is, recovery of a blind child.

Another discovery, however, has emerged: the retinoblastoma is one of the first malignant tumours whose genetic origin has been proven. Its essence is in the genes: not in an oncogene, but in a 'normal' gene. A mutation in the human chromosome 13, acted on by an exogenous carcinogenic agent, switches on the production of a protein causing cell degeneration. When a child inherits a mutation in chromosome 13 from one parent, and when the respective gene from the other parent for unknown reasons does not function, a retinoblastoma occurs. Therefore retinoblastoma is the result of a combination of a gene for malignant degeneration and the absence or non-functioning of a normal gene. If a retino-blastoma gene meets an active, normal gene the disease does not occur. And because the mutation in chromosome 13 can theoretically be found in embryonic cells in the amniotic fluid, there is hope for prenatal diagnosis.

The survival of patients from whom a retinoblastoma has been removed has revealed an even more mysterious genetic horror: at the age of fifteen to seventeen the patients succumb to bone sarcoma, that is, an aggressive cancer of bone cells. These two cancers do not seem to be related. However, the retinoblastoma gene could at the same time be the gene for osteosarcoma. In patients surviving retinoblastoma, this type of bone cancer is 3,000 to 4,000 times more frequent than in the rest of the population. The difference between retinal nerve tissue and bone is so profound that the genetic kinship of the two diseases is one of the great mysteries of disease biology.

And in the individual biology of a particular human being, it looks as though the surgical salvation of a blind child results after twelve years in death, probably from a genetically pre-programmed osteogenic sarcoma.

'Perhaps they'd better . . .' said one of us, when we were reading the report by the molecular geneticist Webster Cavenee. Perhaps they'd better . . . No doubt the aposiopesis was the most terrible thing about this sentence, although the word 'better' was also rather improper and internally unsuitable. Internally, we agreed only with the word 'perhaps'.

This word demonstrates the inappropriateness of medical, in fact I would say general, judgement. More precisely, death sentence. We can, in this sense, make judgements about statistics, not about human beings. More precisely, children.

Science is the art of the soluble, said Peter Medawar.

Science does not reach into the sphere of an insoluble judgement. On the other hand, if there is a solution, that is, a surgically solvable retinoblastoma, it should be solved. And as a rule it will be solved, one of the reasons being that statistics have vents, or tiny openings, and molecular genetics advances so quickly that twelve years is a sufficient period for further developments in the art of the solvable, or at least for simple hope, for the other face of that word 'perhaps'.

And as we were reading Cavanee, leaves were falling from the trees outside, revealing the bare essence of wood, wood that looked sad but was full of vascular bundles distributing vital hormones, no matter how large the sadness or how total the leaf-fall.

And from a distance, from a great and invisible distance, echoed the voices of children who played some game and were cheerful, in spite of everything, in spite of everything distant, great and invisible.

I am not saying this to use lyricism as a cosmetic or a camouflage. I strongly resent lyricism as adhesive tape over the mouth. But there are moments when lyricism still does reach further, beyond the 'better' and the aposiopesis.

Giving Us Heart

Francis Bacon regarded faintheartedness as the greatest obstacle to scientific progress. In the introduction to the *Instauratio Magna* he mentions 'people who are not by longing, nor by hope incensed to penetrate any further'. The pertinent state of mind is defined today as 'but-this-won't-work-anyway' or 'we-can't-afford-that'. In a broader context Ibsen stated that on the ruins of all civilization there will be the inscription, 'He did not dare.'

If 3 December 1967 is remembered, it is as the day Christian Barnard transplanted a human heart for the first time. Although the patient survived only eighteen days, it is the 'He dared' which is remembered in the first place. The technique had been prepared by Shumway and Lower in Stanford; the first clinical transplantation had been performed by Hardy in January 1964, using a chimpanzee heart. The experimental experiences of entire surgical schools were available. But only Barnard dared to trespass both the mystical barrier and the barrier of immunological incompatibility. Maybe he was helped in part by chance, the automobile accident of the heart-donor Derwall (we often accept chances as cosmic winks letting us challenge the barriers and obstacles); maybe he was a little more eager, willing to run a risk and more sure of himself than the others; but, on the whole, he just dared.

Perhaps it may be mentioned that this daring was also endorsed by the progressive success of newer methods of suppressing transplant reactions, that is essentially by another form of daring, one less conspicuous, but with an equally practical and moral meaning. This was the daring to discover induced or acquired immunological tolerance, announced by Billingham, Brent and Medawar in 1944, but published only in 1953 in *Nature*. Its material basis was no bigger than an unborn mouse which was given, while still in the uterus, an injection of cells from another mouse strain and which, once born, would not reject a subsequent skin transplant from the donor strain. It was preceded by something as ignoble as the observations of cattle twins. It was immediately preceded by the first clinical transplantations of kidneys between human twins.

Induced immunological tolerace was a synthetic discovery, that is, as Medawar puts it, an entry into an area so far unknown. Another synthetic discovery was the graft versus host reaction, which remains a serious problem in transplantation. A third synthetic discovery was the proof of the key role and migratory behaviour of lymphocytes. It may be humbly mentioned that Czech immunology was actively present both in the intraembryonic induction of tolerance and in the lymphocyte potentialities story.

And I can say that a synthetic discovery, that is something which can be verified five or ten years later, is an internal drama, situated well below the Shakespearean alternatives of victory or defeat as experienced by a surgeon, and in fact as disquieting as a Beckettian situation where it is not clear who is fighting whom or what.

The synthetic discovery of Medawar's group had broken through a 300-million-year-old history begun by bony fish that could develop cellular transplantation responses. According to Medawar's recollections, 'it gave the decisive audacity to all the biologists and surgeons' who worked on the problem of transplantation of allogenic tissues in mammals and men. And surgeons were quickly ahead of all the others, because it is technically feasible to master all organ transfers, with the exception of brain and testes.

So, with the onset of clinical transplantations, a relation was re-established which T. S. Kuhn had described as no longer operative, namely that technology and praxis brought direct pressure on basic research and leading theories, in the fields of both immunosuppression and immunogenetics. This is typi-fied by the emergence of Cyclosporine A, which was without doubt an analytical and praxis-induced discovery that then led to a renaissance of heart transplants in the 1970s. In science the action often precedes the comprehension, says Karl Popper, and this is very evident in the history of transplan-tations.

But the anniversary and the fact of clinical heart transplan-tations include another essential trait: it was and is a great performance, both in terms of organizational requirements and in terms of heart mythology. It is conspicuous, it is the arrival of medicine on the lunar surface: not that other performances and results do not deserve a similar attention and admiration, but that this performance was as exposed and visible as Neil Armstrong's historical step. In this sense its psychological light falls on the whole field and on all hospital beds and laboratory tables and we can say that even the routine examination of the transplant patient's lymphocytes feels different because they are from one of 'the hearts'. And this is true when the scrutiny does not aim at a synthetic discovery, which is harder to make nowadays and needs more and more equipment and organization.

The moral relevance of transplants is, of course, more

conspicuous in circumstances where the overcoming of organ-
izational and other rather external difficulties is unduly com-
plicated. It is a clear answer to all the 'but-it-won't-work-
anyways' and 'we-couldn't-afford-thats' of a delayed and
lagging society.

What Barnard dared to do decades ago can be described as
giving us all heart in the broadest metaphorical sense, and over
all the world.

In reality the transplant procedure looks of course (like
everything with a broad sense and effect) very plain, routine
and quiet. Under quiet spotlights, calm figures cover with
drapes the cooled, hypothermic body of the recipient, which
looks like something orphan-like, excluded, primary as an
Adam. They work their way with knives and saws to the old
heart, they detour the blood to the extracorporeal circulation
with cannulae, and the heart, its coronaries still supplied with
blood but otherwise jobless and beating lightly and delibera-
tely, is lifted with claw-like forceps, detached in the atrium and
the aorta, so that the pericardium is empty with an unbeliev-
able cosmic emptiness expanding in time. The instruments
click and ping. Quietly spoken orders hover over the body that
dreams under the sheets that it is morning and that it is
brushing its teeth. The new heart is brought in the melting
crushed ice. In a distant corner of the theatre two nurses chat.
Atrium to atrium and aorta to aorta are being sewn, the new
heart is awakened to new life by electric shocks, evacuated of
air by needle punctures, the fourth hour is passing, the blood is
let back into its historical limits, which will be again called the
living human body, the quiet battlefield is taken over by the
assistant, the bloody green gowns are thrown on the tiles of the
anteroom and in the main room the waves of EKG, of
oesophageal temperature, of systolic and diastolic pressure

and central venous pressure run on the screen — after the fashion of the last four million years.

Only it is based not on twenty, but on sixty and more years of accumulated knowledge and skills.

I have experienced an analogous peace on Kitt Peak in Arizona, where telescopes and computers, under the shining white domes of the observatories, look for the symmetric pairs of galaxies and paired chains of galaxies which would be a proof that the cosmic strings, the hypothetical remnants of the Big Bang, really exist and run on above our beating hearts.

The Emperor Inside Out

Once he replied: 'You wrote to me, "This is not possible," but that's not French.'

Goethe said about him to Eckermann: 'He was Somebody and one could see that he was Somebody.' 'He was demoniac through and through.' Goethe should have known because he had met the man and talked to him about *The Sorrows of Young Werther* and the conversation had been more like a prosecutor's case against the defendant Werther. Goethe also said about him: 'In his personality there was superiority. But, most of all, people were convinced that with him they would get somewhere.'

Goethe also said about him, seven years after his death:

> He was one of the most creative people ever to have lived; there is also the creativity of deeds, and that, in many cases, stands even higher . . . Whether a man proves his genius in science . . . or in the administration of the state . . . makes no difference, what matters is whether the idea, the discovery, or the deed are alive, and whether they are able to live on . . .

But the best thing Goethe said — and this probably applies to many who are powerful through their descent, their will or their destiny — was that 'Napoleon was particularly great in that at every hour he was the same. Before a battle, during a battle, after a battle, after victory, after defeat . . . he always knew clearly what he had to do. He was always in his element.'

Goethe had his own affinity with the powerful and he talked of Napoleon virtually every minute, attributing his amazing strength to his health: that Napoleon was the second son of an eighteen-year-old mother was, in Goethe's theory of health, a guarantee of an exceptional condition in the child; the youngest of the Bonaparte couple's eight children was thus, according to Goethe's ideas, the weakest.

Theories of health are sometimes fallacious, especially the poetical ones. The youngest child, Jerome, was in fact, along with Joseph, the only one who did not suffer from a stomach disorder which ran in the family. His sister Elise showed signs of stomach ulcers, as did Pauline; Caroline died of something that was probably a stomach cancer and much the same happened to brother Lucien and possibly also to Louis. Napoleon's grandfather, Joseph Bonaparte, and his great-uncle Charles, as well as his sister Gertrude, died of constriction of the pylorus, with a tumour (proved by autopsy) in the region of the stomach. Charles, in addition, had hard nodules in the pancreas, which may also have originated from tumours. This inherited affliction was the subject of a study by Vasseur (1926) and it is also in agreement with P. Hillemand's pathology of Napoleon (1970). Napoleon, according to the relatively accurate account of the post-mortem performed by his Corsican doctor Antonmarchi on the island of St Helena in May 1821, had a perforated stomach ulcer located 'to the right of the tumour mass'.

The fact is that Napoleon had suffered from stomach cramps since at least 1802; these would come on a few hours after eating and were usually accompanied by vomiting. Sometimes they could be assuaged by a light snack. The

Brigade General, the victor of Toulon, the victor of Monte-notte, Dega, Millesima and Arcolle, the commander-in-chief of the campaign in Egypt, the victor of Marengo, from 1799 First Consul, then Life Consul, and two years later the Emperor Napoleon I, that short, thin, totally self-assured and indomitably resolute first man in Europe, the man who 'always knows what he had to do and is always in his element', was secretly writhing in pain, sleeping for his customary four hours with the prospect of a further attack, in the event of which a light meal was invariably standing ready by his bedside; at two o'clock in the morning he regularly ate 'chocolate or ice-cream'. At Austerlitz, at Wagram and on the Berezina, as well as at international negotiations, when he planted his relations and generals upon new and ancient thrones, when he became Protector of the Rhenish League and King of Italy, he would carry in the pockets of his dark-green uniform some ridiculous little biscuits and aniseed or liquorice twists and swallow them whenever an attack came. He was tormented by particularly cruel pain during the Battle of Leipzig, which incidentally he lost, whereas what excruciated him at Waterloo seems to have been haemorrhoids, to such an extent that he could not bear to stay in the saddle. From childhood on he'd had difficulties with urinating. Sometimes he would faint – the most plausible explanation of which is a hypoglycaemic crisis – and he had festering skin diseases, running sores first described as nettle-rash and later as chronic prurigo.

All these troubles got worse when, after Moscow, his progressive decline began. Nevertheless, they probably had no effect on the destiny, the general destiny as it were, of the man from whose vocabulary the words 'this is not possible' were missing. When assessing the wheel of history we do not look at itches or the stomach.

After 1810, however, something new happened, something that could not be overcome like that personal Waterloo, something that got inside him, as he himself described his disease, which he regarded as cancer. From that time on a process clearly began which the emperor of his own inside could not master because he was gradually losing himself. The Emperor was steadily getting fatter, to the point of downright obesity in the years of St Helena; he was losing his decisiveness and will-power; he had attacks of somnolence and lethargy. As early as May 1810, he actually fell asleep during a ball, while sitting on the throne. The elegance of his demeanour went, together with the sharp features of his face. Gone was his presence of mind. The Emperor was literally disintegrating. This was how Antonmarchi saw him after 1815: 'beautiful hands, rounded breasts, his skin white and delicate, no fine hair, maybe only [not specified by Antonmarchi] Any beautiful lady might be proud of that chest . . .' Napoleon's sexual behaviour changed to such an extent that Richardson in his monograph was able to refer to the bisexual Emperor and prisoner on St Helena (1972). The post-mortem established a remarkable atrophy of his sex organs.

Thus, at the time of the fall of Paris in 1814, on Elba, during the final Hundred Days of the empire and at Waterloo, he was no longer the one who was always the same; he was merely one who, whipped up by circumstances, inertia and the remnants of his will-power, forced himself to be his own memory. That which died on St Helena was merely the obese shadow of the Emperor, a shadow who at least insisted on a dark-green uniform now that his old one was too tight, faded and shabby. And because the appropriate green cloth was not to be found on the island, only a material with a touch of yellow in it, and because Napoleon obstinately refused it, the matter was eventually settled – according to the testimony of Hudson Lowe, the Governor – by having the old uniform unpicked at the seams, underlaid and turned inside out.

One of the most powerful men in history, then, was eventually all inside out, except for those buttons. The man who had been in command of a continent and of his own internal Waterloo was finally caught in the counter-movement of the wheel of his disease, the victim of his pituitary.

Hillemand himself comes out in favour of a tumour of the pituitary and concludes that:

> it was the neuroendocrinological syndrome of his final twelve years that played the decisive role in the destinies of the Empire and of France. An overstimulated imagination and misguided ambitions, no longer controlled by his keen judgement, a weakening of his will, sometimes masked by fits of obstinacy, his hesitancy, sleepiness, physical fatigue – these were the main causes of his downfall.

P. Rentchnik (1977) is the first to introduce into Napoleon's pathology the Zollinger–Ellison syndrome, in which multiple small tumours, situated as a rule in the pancreas, secrete the hormone gastrin, which causes an increased production and acidity of the stomach juice and thereby repeated and obstinate ulcers of the stomach and the duodenum. In one-quarter of all patients, however, gastrinoma is part of a multiple endocrinological adenomatosis (MEA) of type 1, which is a sex-linked disease with a high penetration, that is with a large number of individuals displaying clinical phenomena of a genetically linked anomaly. Persons with MEA 1 have tumours, sometimes even malignant ones, affecting the parathyroid glands, the pancreatic islands and the pituitary. This may result in secondary kidney disorder, increasing insulin production causing hypoglycaemic conditions (reduction in the blood-sugar level), reduced thyroid function with obesity, fatigue, drowsiness, whiteness of skin, loss of skin hair, atrophy of the genitals and adrenal insufficiency exhibited in situations of stress. These and other symptoms are mutually interlinked in a complex manner, so that for each consequence, for example obesity, a number of causes may be listed.

In the history of diseases and diseases in history nothing is certain and a lot of things are possible, yet it would seem that there was no need for anyone to poison what was left of the Emperor on St Helena – even though, given the circumstances, arsenic might well be expected. On the contrary, out of the fifty-two years of his life the man probably spent a good half overcoming his multiple afflictions – afflictions against which he could mobilize neither his Code Napoléon nor his Continental Blockade and to whose final breakthrough he actually succumbed later than might have been expected. His political and military retreat was, by a tragic irony of fate, in step with the disintegration of his personality. The military actions of the Napoleonic Wars showed a previously unparalleled effectiveness in terms of loss of life. This historical pathology thus, with its own tragic irony, runs parallel to the endocrinologic pathology of the Emperor, who long before his death had lost himself.

The Statue

The huge statue in the Lincoln Memorial at Washington radiates serenity, nobleness and dignified kindheartedness. The elongated head, rimmed by a beard and receding hair, is turned to the entrance, and from underneath the heavy eyelids it watches the minuscule figures of visitors who climb the stairs and walk among the massive Doric columns, to stand in absolute silence in the open space of this semi-temple. The statue, by its very essence, discourages the tourists from the usual scurrying and murmuring. The statue visibly thinks. Its thoughts seem to bring back the tens of thousands of dead from the Civil War, the first total war in modern history. Lincoln worked to terminate the conflict just as urgently as he insisted on preserving the Union. Five days after General Lee surrendered to Grant at Appomattox, and a couple of days after the President gave a talking-to to the hard-boiled General Sherman ('Out of all the men I have ever met, he had the most traits of greatness combined with goodness,' wrote Sherman later), Abraham Lincoln was shot by the actor John Wilkes Booth in the box of the Ford Theater in Washington.

The statue seems to remember even that moment at 10.13 p.m., on 14 April 1865, when Booth, unchecked, slipped into the President's box, barred the door with a latch he had prepared, and shot Lincoln – sitting in his rocking chair, at a moment when he was turning in the opposite direction, as if someone from the audience called — from the distance of half a metre, in the left side of his nape.

The statue recalls this moment with supreme composure; throughout his term, the President dreamed about being assassinated, believed his dreams and accepted them with fatalistic resignation. He refused bodyguards: maybe that is why no one was guarding the box at the critical moment, so that Booth even managed to slash Major Rathbone, who was also present. While climbing over the balustrade to the stage, where the actors were standing motionless, Booth got his leg tangled in the flag, dropped on the other leg, broke it, and, watched by the audience, stumbled backstage, waving his knife and shouting, '*Sic semper tryannis!*' In the meantime an army doctor, the first man to reach the box, restored the President's breathing and pulse by artificial respiration, found the wound and removed blood clots with his fingers. Lincoln was carried to the house next door, the wound was repeatedly probed with non-sterile probes, which failed to locate the bullet in the brain, and life was preserved until the following morning: Lincoln died at 7.22 a.m. Even modern technical facilities would have been of little help.

One of the ironies of history is that the autopsy document and other medical records dating from 15 April are contradictory in describing where in the brain the bullet lodged and for a hundred years it was not clear what had caused bone fractures in the ceiling of both eye orbits, or even what the exact mechanism of death was. The role of Booth, his own death and his possible associates, will remain a mystery for ever. Oddly enough, the fatal shot had a trajectory not dissimilar from the shot that killed President Kennedy.

Sadness can also be detected in the statue's great calmness. From the age of thirty, Lincoln suffered from attacks of extreme melancholia accompanied by delirium. In a letter written in 1841, when he was thirty-two, he says he must change, or die. The son of a lumberman, he was never close to his father, lost his mother at nine, and led a more or less solitary and haphazard life in the relative wilderness of northern Illinois: he built log cabins, chased wolves, kept bees, and once he even gathered volunteers to fight the Indians, which – just like his strength – won him some fame in his neighbourhood. His figure attracted attention; besides his very negligent way of dressing, it was mainly his 193 cm of height. He was a big scarecrow with a hollow chest, drooping shoulders, unusually long shins and gigantic feet. His hands were elongated and graceful, with spider-like fingers.

The statue in the memorial sits in a chair and looks down, the head slightly bent; the hands lie on the arms of the chair, the fingers of the right hand loose, those of the left hand clenched in a fist. The sculptor, D. C. French, has preserved all of the features without accentuating the peculiarities. It is evident from photographs that Lincoln's shins were so long that in the sitting position his knees were much higher that his pelvis. Standing up he produced such a towering impression that in one war photograph, in front of army tents and surrounded by thirteen high-ranking officers, he looks like an embarrassed teacher, in top hat and tails, among teenage pupils shorter by a head. Even the respectful soldiers of the Union Army talked about how extremely comical Lincoln looked on horseback: his legs somehow got entangled with the legs of the horse, and while he was getting on the horse his arms looked 'like the hind legs of a locust'. His pale, greyish eyes were covered by drooping eyelids; he was extremely far-sighted and squinted.

Lincoln recovered from his acute melancholia after he

married in 1842; he reached a sort of good-natured equilibrium and faced his tasks with robust seriousness. On the advice of his followers, he took up law studies and graduated, though he tired easily and did not manage to read more than two or three pages at a time; he had the rest read to him. In the political arena, he bore everything with resignation and singularly moderate humour. He was incapable of rhetorical improvisation, but filled his written speeches with a straightforward wisdom that is still quoted. However, even as President he gave an impression of permanent exhaustion: 'as he walked, melancholy was dripping from him,' in the words of a contemporary. He had to cope with his own people's hatred; for instance, Stanton described him as the gorilla and ape from Illinois, visited by fits of 'pitiful dumbness'. He had to bear his personal tragedies, illnesses and the deaths of sons; eventually he even had to become a general among generals and overcome the biggest crisis in the history of the United States.

He managed to win, maintain the Union and contribute to the liberation of the slaves, even if his murderer regarded himself as the executor of a tyrant, and although Lincoln himself thought more about the casualities than about the victory.

Thirty-one years after Lincoln's death the French paediatrician Marfan described a hereditary anomaly based on a disorganization of connective tissues, affecting at least one out of three systems, the skeleton, the eyes, and the heart and blood vessels. In 1964, the American H. Schwartz published a study mentioning traits in Lincoln's genealogy that would attest a disposition for Marfan's syndrome. Starting with Mordecai Lincoln, born in 1686, exterior morphological signs of the syndrome were found in thirteen men in two branches of the family, while a fully developed syndrome was proved by

Schwartz both in the President and in a boy from the ninth generation of the second family branch, a boy he had personally examined. The syndrome was probably also developed in three of the President's sons, demonstrating a marked psychiatric symptomatology, defined by P. Bieler as imbecility in one case and oligophreny in the second and third cases. According to most psychiatric textbooks, mental retardation in Marfan's syndrome is relatively restrained; Schwartz also cites reports of high intelligence related to the syndrome.

The skeletal modifications can be denoted as unproportional elongation of some bones: in Lincoln's case they fully fall within the quantitative limits set for Marfan's syndrome. Data about his arms' span are not available, but Schwartz makes do with the fact that the span was abnormal. During a military parade in Maine, Lincoln noted: 'I do not believe anyone in this regiment has longer arms than I have.' On plaster casts of Lincoln's hands, the sculptor Bartlett measured the first segment of the middle finger and found it to be 12 mm longer than the segment of a normal hand; the bones were generally gracile, the muscles thin, the joints loose. A clenched fist corresponded to the notion of arachnodactylia, or spider-like fingers. The left arm was longer than the right one, although Lincoln was right-handed, but the thumb of the left hand was 10 mm shorter than the thumb of the right hand.

In the eyes the deviation from the standard was such (+ 6.75 diopters) that it could not possibly be an acquired defect (M. H. Shutes, 1957). Lincoln's father was blind in one eye and one of Lincoln's sons had very weak eyesight in addition to suffering from vertical squinting; this son died of heart failure at eighteen, which seems to confirm the hereditary disease of the cardiovascular system.

All this supports hereditary Marfan's syndrome, probably

connected with a deviation in the pituitary gland. This is undoubtedly a safer diagnosis than that of a political and cerebral cause of death. The establishment of a safe diagnosis of such a syndrome certainly does not follow the usual historical path of celebrating the celebrities, nor is it within the boundaries of historically acceptable ailments of great men, which include mainly diseases of the heart and lungs, exhaustion from statesmanship and wounds inflicted in battles, and, at the extreme, endocrinologic deviations and deformations of body and personality. It appears, however, that this diagnosis does not spoil anyone's fun either.

In any case, the statue in the Lincoln Memorial is also a six-metre-tall marble monument of the external symptoms of Marfan's syndrome. Not many of our syndromes get such a statue. Not many of us, despite all syndromes, get to be Lincolns.

Pedestrians and Cells

From an aerial view a street filled with pedestrians is not unlike a blood vessel in a microcinematographic recording and a square is not unlike the area of an inflammation on a mesothelial membrane, where leucocytes pick their way among attractions such as activated components of complement, products of disintegrated cells and bacterial substances, while more or less obeying intercellular memoranda called lymphokines or cytokines. According to Bessis, their speed rate at a temperature of 37°C ranges between nineteen to forty microns per minute, that is, a couple of centimetres per day, a distance they rarely cover, just as there is no record of a town pedestrian covering 60 kilometres in one day.

There are, however, other similarities. Cells move at a speed directly dependent on the temperature of the environment. Pedestrians in a town move at a speed directly dependent on the size of the town, more precisely according to an equation establishing that the average velocity of a solitary walker, in feet per second, equals the constant 0.05 plus 0.86 multiplied by the logarithm of the number of inhabitants, that is $V = 0.05 + 0.86 \, (\log P)$. This dependence was discovered by M. H. Bornstein and H. G. Bornstein (*Nature*, 259:557, 1976) when they measured the speed of twenty incidental pedestrians in fifteen towns of six European, Asian and North American countries on a sunny, dry day in the main artery of the town, by recording the time necessary to cover the distance of 50 feet.

They marked the distance on the pavement by chalk and, unseen, registered the motility of pedestrians who had no obstacles in their way, were not chased by anyone, did not carry too much, and were not visibly decrepit. Which shows how much easier it is for psychologist–behaviourists to do their job than for cell researchers.

The happy behaviourist Bornstein discovered that in the town of Psychro in Crete (365 inhabitants), 50 feet were covered in 18.1 plus/minus 4.1 seconds; in Corte, France (5,491 inhabitants), in 15.1 plus/minus 1.8 seconds; in Safed, Israel (14,000 inhabitants), in 13.5 plus/minus 2.5 seconds; in New Haven, Connecticut (138,000 inhabitants), in 11.4 plus/minus 1.8 seconds; and in Munich, West Germany (1,340,000 inhabitants), in 8.9 plus/minus 1.3 seconds, etc.

Nevertheless, we Czechs have a special relationship with the linear dependence calculated from all fifteen town measurements. The city with the most marked deviation from the straight line of linear regression towards a higher velocity of walking was Prague, specifically Wenceslas Square. That is where the highest speed rate of walking was registered – 50 feet in 8.5 plus/minus 1.3 seconds, with a population of 1,092,759.

Without intending to joke – like Harold Morowitz, who calculated that according to the Bornsteins' equation Robinson Crusoe and Friday would have had to walk at an average speed of 6 metres per minute, and Thoreau at his pond in Walden at a speed of 90 cm per minute, a demanding task even for a philosopher deep in thought – let us note that the speed of inhabitants in another Czech city, Brno, 10.4 plus/minus 1.8 seconds for 50 feet with the number of inhabitants amounting to 341,948 (data from 1974), corresponded to the formula, and that only in Prague do we seem to be particularly overburdened by social stimuli and want to get the hell out of Wenceslas Square at a speed unusual for other places and unconditioned by the Czech and Moravian genetic make-up.

And here we are justified, biologically and psychologically, in adding that we do not know anyone who would go to Wenceslas Square to flee from stimuli, that the percentage of pedestrians who either live or hold jobs there must be negligible, certainly zero in a sample of twenty pedestrians; and that our velocity in the given locality is accelerated mainly by the expectancy and occurrence of shopping stimuli or even cultural stimuli. The 'social and physical environment' quoted in the report under discussion has a direct impact on individual behaviour in Prague as well, although the mechanisms differ grossly from the mechanisms of moving around in a street in Heraklion, Crete, or on Flatbush Avenue in Brooklyn, New York. While it is difficult to spot a pedestrain hunting for a dumpling mix on Flatbush Avenue, you do not see, on a sunny day in Wenceslas Square, groups of vigorous young men who ask you with a sharp smile for a contribution to increase their standard of living. Consequently, you quicken your pace quite substantially. Their own sluggish movement contributes to a lower motility than the one calculated in the Bornsteins' formula. The only explanation for the difference between the Prague and Brno motilities must be sought in the existence of the equestrian statue of St Wenceslas in the Prague square. Statues haunting pedestrians in daylight constitute a novel type of stimulation unknown to sociobiology.

It seems we either crawl or dash according to the formula anywhere in the world, although in reality, in the lives of specific individuals, the driving forces and movements are totally different, frequently incommensurable and notably obscure.

One can snigger at the customs of behaviourists. But it must be admitted that in biology we are also controlled by such customs, and that our descriptions of the behaviour of cells on mesothelial membranes and in allogenic grafts, no matter whether inspired by impressions from microcinematographic recordings or by capturing molecular signs and signals, are at best a certain kind of cellular behaviourism.

Only the poor cells cannot comment.

However, the distance between the measured speed of a citizen walking between two chalk marks in the business centre of a town and the mind of that same citizen is a distance that must be covered in learning about the cells which exist and function and walk in the basis and background of all our healths and sicknesses.

All the same, I'd like to know why here in Prague we're all in such a hurry.

A Walk in the Forest

This was a walk with a beautiful young lady who looked Indian and had mastered the art of attentive listening. Forests in the presence of such personalities are much deeper and more meaningful than otherwise.

It was snowing. The forest recalled a primeval forest and the twilight a primeval night. An oldish man with gentle eyes, in fur cap and voluminous slippers, was standing between a chicken coop and a rabbit hutch. He was talking to his slice of agriculture, as such men are in the habit of doing. On our greeting him, he came up and began a conversation.

Would we accept advice? Yes, gladly. Do we know that good returns? No, we don't. But it does, he said, it comes to the head of the bed at dusk. Yes, it returns to the feet in the morning. It comes back in bread and in water and in the word of the law.

And did we know that the road to the light is open? One has only to repent one's evil deeds, errors and trickery; one has only to ask after the meaning of things, to reflect earnestly and unyieldingly, and then the Thought will watch over us and the light will rise at the end of every journey.

Then he told us about the man who heard the voice of Justice when he was in the lavatory, since elsewhere he felt ashamed to listen to the voice of Justice.

Then he told us of his sons, who had gone astray, except for one who still visited him, although he was deserted and alone and the road through the forest was hardly passable for a motor vehicle.

Then he showed us the way to the main road and followed us with weakly shining eyes.

Then he disappeared in the dusk.

We took the view on the one hand that his was a pleasant form of mild schizophrenia. Besides, any kind of mild schizophrenia is more pleasant in the woods than in a tram or in the household.

On the other hand, we took the view that if we met Francisco Pizarro in the forest, when he had just packed up the Incas' treasure, tortured the King, Atahualpa, and murdered 10,000 subjects, we would very likely consider him the normal Francisco Pizarro. That if we met Francisco de Benalcazar, who, drunk, had all the Indian officials in Quito slowly roasted over a fire, we would consider him the quite normal Francisco de Benalcazar, slightly disoriented in geography.

But a man with a gentle eye, in capacious slippers, and humbly meditating on good and evil, a man who on meeting people in the forest twilight wishes to give advice, appears nutty as a fruitcake.

We concluded that, though the diagnosis was correct, the error was ours and, when the main road showed among the trees, we reflected earnestly and unyieldingly on the meaning of things.

And it was apparent to us that it was a very old road, linking Cuzco and Sachahuaman, while further to the south-east we could hear the murmur of the great lake Titicaca, and the melting of the widespread snow.

My professor of psychiatry, one of the great personalities who vanished in the last few decades in the heart of Europe, looked like an overgrown Charlie Chaplin with a Cyrano-like beard and funny black jacket. He used to open his lectures with a statement delivered from the very front of the platform: 'Dear colleagues, the greatest problem of psychiatry is the problem of normality. Look, for instance, at me. And I am going to teach you psychiatry, anyway.'

He was one of the few really normal, healthy, impressive persons I have met in my life. He even gave me an A in pharmacology, standing in for the pharmacology professor and with me standing in as a student who was interested in sedatives and painkillers.

After him, I have met and worked with such an impressive number of alcoholics, paranoiacs and pre-senile psychotics that I have to ask, Who was and who is normal under the conditions of the present world? I would love to see a Who's Who in the World of Sanity and I would love to see a Who's Who of Sanity for the First World, the Second World and the Third World, because an Idi Amin, say, may be normal in the south, and more or less paranoid schizophrenic in the north.

By what standards was Atahualpa normal and Pizarro mad and vice versa?

With all this in mind, I must reiterate that in the forest and under those conditions we had a reassuring talk with a sound and healthy schizophrenic.

Men with Knives

It is no doubt horrible, but even large animals, in many aspects unpleasantly similar to man, must be killed in large numbers. So there must be people who daily face the animals' mortal anguish, their desperate desire to escape, their last struggle. What can these people's relationship to nature be, nature that is the object of loving care and protection by law? And what can these people's relationship to certain internal matters of nature be, such as the evocation of death, the shedding of blood and the causing of pain, things which are essentially taboo in a cultural society?

A slaughterhouse is a nocturnal and subterranean consciousness of the city, which needs and demands animal proteins for the purpose of a healthy development of young and old generations on the one hand, but on the other hand turns away in disgust from the smell of blood, intestinal action and reflexive spasms of the muscles. For a decent man, the mortal spasms, no matter what we call them, are acceptable in flies, mice, chickens and fish, but are unacceptable in large mammals with dark knowing eyes, or very sad eyes. Blood is tolerable in wipable drops on the kitchen table, not in puddles and lakes on a concrete floor.

'I couldn't do it,' says the decent man.

The decent man also faints in an autopsy room, and sophisticated individuals collapse even in operating theatres.

The moral codex, delimited by the phrase 'I-couldn't-do-it' and by fainting, is of course a Tartuffian moral codex.

And the Tartuffian city absorbs with great interest artistic representations of the destruction of enemy troops, and prettified reactions to a shot in the chest or the liver in detective stories. Weaned on these cultural ways of death, it believes that cattle (pieces of beef) falling at five-minute intervals in a place full of muffled blows, mooing and screeching and black steaming streams, can be a line of work only for the jaded, the drunk, the different, the ostracized, for occasional sadists and similar individuals.

However, this work is simply work of men with knives.

The men with knives undoubtedly differ from the views of the fainting public. All men with knives do. From the evolutionary point of view, it is difficult to say what they are different from. They were not different in the time of hunters and shepherds; and even today they are not different from many ethnic groups sharing this planet with the fainting public. On the contrary, once a year, various so-called aborigines hold collective feasts, when whole villages gather at neighbourly manifestations, something like the Corpus Christi ceremony and similar rituals, and they slaughter herds of buffaloes or capybara or seals or antelope or peccaries, using methods next to which conveyor belts with pigs doped by carbon dioxide seem very gentle facilities. (It cannot be said, however, that slaughterhouse technology has progressed proportionally to other fields of industrial activity. We probably do not take those domestic animals, man's friends, or those men with knives, too much to heart.)

In view of the above-mentioned aboriginal ceremonies, I venture to think that it is not the men with the knives who are different, but the fainting public, which, within the bounds of technological civilization, has invented other diversions and has closed off the meat-processing industry in more or less hygienic and more or less well-controlled enclaves, from which, moreover, the Tartuffian moral codex requires invisibility.

Therefore I would not describe the relationship of the men with knives towards nature as different; if you'll excuse me, I would describe it as a primary relationship. The men with knives exemplify the division in approaches to nature — namely, the passive pastoral approach of the fainting public, and the exploiting, dramatic and militant approach, where it has never been possible to establish taboos which are regarded otherwise as the foundation of culture in nations with advanced civilization.

The man with a knife is of course psychologically conditioned by the taboos of an advanced culture. As a beginner in the meat industry he is not asked to slaughter young animals; he has to overcome all kinds of uneasy feelings and often arrives at a sense of manly superiority, probably not without risk. But later he settles in a professional unseeing and unhearing, sharply delimited by the walls of slaughterhouse and untransferable into so-called civilian life. I have heard many biographies of slaughterhouse employees, emphasized with conspicuous selectivity, who in their leisure time were veritable believers in pastoral nature and delicate relationships, probably by way of compensation. I have also heard of various alcoholic curriculae, but I cannot even start listing the professions in which such curriculae are more frequent; there isn't room.

Professional breaking of taboos in a society is usually not the cause of individual aberration and breakdown. There might be a selective mechanism for men who can do 'it', but there is no universal professional deformity. There is no universal addiction to blood, either in prosecutors, or surgeons, or butchers. There are perhaps certain idiosyncrasies cultivated by respective professions. It is butchers and doctors who are the most agitated by the prospect of local anaesthetic in a dentist's chair. Blood seen on a highway has the same emotional impact on a butcher, an experienced surgeon and a layman. It was not the butcher who used to kill newborn kittens at our place; he felt sick at the idea. It was the virtuous housewife.

Because kittens are killed, while animals in slaughterhouses are slaughtered. That is the core of the problem. There is no one who kills fifty cows or pigs in a shift. There are only the men in a slaughterhouse, the men wielding a hammer and a stun gun, which can be too weak for some bulls' skulls, the men tying up the hind legs, the men cutting throats. Subjectively, they carry out something like the destruction of enemy troops, only they get no medals.

The men with knives, having taken off their working overalls and having left the walls of the slaughterhouse, become the men in the street or the men in nature, and how they will behave depends more on the general character of the street and the general state of the collective aesthetic and moral feeling. I still have the feeling that because of the heart of the matter they must know more than the fainting public. They know what they do not do, they know what they can do.

And it is undoubtedly a rather mythical profession, although one cannot expect every butcher to become Abel Tiffauges from Tournier's novel *Le Roi des Aulnes* (1970); in this giant and potentially fascist 'cannibal', the snare of the body, blood and inferiority merge in a gigantic myth – 'When I say "I like meat, I like blood, I like carnality," what matters is the verb "like".'

But even Abel Tiffauges's destiny was determined by public history. The point of public history is, basically, to confine the notion of the man with the knife within the most narrow technological boundaries, perhaps in the area of a private myth, and not to allow it to get the upper hand. Never. Nowhere.

The World in Miniature

Most human urges can be described as a tendency to have something, anything, at home. There are some people so dextrous that they are able to build models of the Pyramids or the Santa Maria or the scene in Bethlehem (that affair with the star and some kings) or streetcars or the Tower of Pisa or a kitchen or a parlour or any one of hundreds of other popular relics out of toothpicks or cardboard and maybe a little glue. There are some who can even make their models move, and they sometimes get written up in their local newspapers, or else their work is sent to exhibitions far away. There are still other folk who don't desire relics, but who love the wonders of technology. These people build (with the aid of fancy machined metals and electric gismos) models of jumbo jets, or fully automated trains with tunnels and brightly lit switchyards, or racing tracks for formula one cars, or factories and highways, or else some sort of big military equipment. They occasionally even have conventions where the builders of model aeroplanes demonstrate and trade their fancy creations.

Some of these models are so popular that the toy industry has developed a selection of kits that provide ready-to-assemble versions of cars or jets, so that the less talented of us can do the same thing, only a bit more expensively.

I don't know a man alive who isn't overcome by an uncontrollable interest when he sees such a carefully assembled model, even though he sees the real thing all the time. Hardly anyone will stand to enjoy the beauty of a town square – the magic of all the moving pedestrians and historical clocks, the colourful cars struggling with signs and commands – but everyone is willing to stand for hours at a model of the same thing and admire the miracle it worked, even though in real life it is often a miracle as well.

I therefore conclude that the miniaturization of the world we live in is an instinctive act, the realization of an underlying urge to bring the large things outside into our friendly little spaces inside. There's something about controlling large things through the reduction of space and time; a miniaturization which is on the fringes of the possibilities of our fingers, but fully within the realm of our feelings for beauty and permanence. And it isn't just some simple childish instinct either, nor is it simply playing. On the contrary: the child who builds a zoo or a railroad or a little town out of cardboard in a corner has simply been granted the chance to realize that general human desire which adults (who have lost the privilege of leisure) largely cannot realize.

Perhaps, to our perceptions, the outside world is, for some reason, a little too big for us; it has grown somehow over our heads. In miniature models, there are no faulty connections, no unkept airline schedules, no dangerous speeds, no crashes of jumbo jets, nor even fires or detours. In the miniature world, everything functions. Everything is simply as it ought to be.

And, in essence, the scientist who models the incomprehensible complexity and scope of organic and inorganic processes in a clever little experiment, and who then presents a paper about his findings (which is nothing more than a miniature excerpt of the terrible denouement of events) is himself quite

like the builder of miniature railroads in miniature land-
scapes. Indeed, so is the artist, who gives a little version of the
state of things in several colours, several notes or several
verses.

At bottom, the joy of a completed miniature is the same for
people from all walks of life, even though they may call it by
different names. And it's only the strange names that make
scientific and artistic joys seem less understandable.

Last but not least, there are basic structures which can be
established with coarse measurements and then repeated in
ever finer and finer measurements, which of course will result
in greater and greater value for the outline of the given
geometric formations. The relation of two neighbouring (sub-
sequent) measurements is constant for all scales used. The
natural objects having this quality are said to have self-
symmetry, and are denoted by Mandelbrot as fractals. All of
us, well experienced since infancy in natural forms, have in our
instincts, bred in the bone so to speak, a feeling for possible
structures in both directions, upwards, into the supravisible,
and downwards, into the infravisible (called invisible). We
have a sort of *a priori* quasi-intuitive sense of how this tussock
will grow, how these cells will aggregate, how this focus of
necrotizing inflammation will look, how this ant-hill will
enlarge. And this sense can be modelled by means of the
fractals with a satisfying exactness.

I suggest that the pleasure we take in miniaturization (and,
on the other side, in enlarging into graspable and understand-
able sizes) has, in addition to playfulness, this relatively
sublime basis, and that we are in a way sensually and
imaginatively prepared for the newly generated artefacts
constituted in the beautiful computer models of Mandelbrot's
sets.

[79]

In the model of the Santa Maria we have the discovery of America in a manageable scale and at home. In Mandelbrot's sets we have the structure of nature from leucocytes to stars, at home and in a manageable form of the terrifying.

Visible Microbes

There are pictures in our lab, put up to cheer the eye, of various mythical monsters: Cerberus, the Harpies, Chimeras and the giant Polyphemus, who is squeezing Ulysses in his fist like a B lymphocyte and who reminds one of a well-known scientist. We also have a poster that says, 'Don't be afraid of insects. They can't help looking stupid.' The insects in the picture don't remind one of anything. They really don't look too good.

Insects have never reminded people of anything but other insects, which naturally arouses curiosity at every encounter of the first to third kind. It's like meeting ET, except very much in the plural.

I recently had an encounter near a forest that seemed to be mostly composed of stinging nettles. It was with a nest or loose cocoon of caterpillars of the Peacock butterfly, a horde of tiny gremlin-like creatures. Sitting there among their fibres, they probably got a little scared. They tried to deter my closer approach by pulsating the fronts of their tiny bodies, beat–beat. I wouldn't mind that so much, but the beat–beat was uncannily accurate, at intervals of about a second and a half, and what's more it took the form of a wave: one of them in the front started it and it then went through the whole nest, as if there were a single cardiac muscle at work. When it came to an end there was a pause of a second or so and then the conductor in the front began another one. Even if I assume the possibility of a time coupling in the entire nest/cocoon, the transfer of the impulse from the front to the back, controlled either by the caterpillars' eyes or by some pheromone, there is still the utter mystery of the first caterpillar, who started each wave and who could scarcely see it complete itself at the back. I was seized by such curiosity that I've been asking entomologists about it ever since, but so far to no avail.

And that is what insects are like, all the time. They are mysterious. And they do not look good.

Not to look good from the human point of view seems to be the insects' universal quality; if one of them appears elegant to the naked eye, then just look at its hairy body or mandibular head through a magnifying glass. By their shapes and behaviour insects look to me like microbes, magnified a thousand or ten thousand times. If the microbes' salami-like or doughnut-shaped bodies, with their fimbria, cilia or flagella, could be measured in centimetres instead of microns and could walk around on a table, following some chemotactic stimuli, the effect would be conspicuously similar to the passage of the Gypsy Moth caterpillars or to the movement of adult specimens of absurdly and prehistorically wax-plated scale insects, deafened and dazed by pheromone signals or scents. The movement of the flagella might resemble the beating of my caterpillars. As for that one who started the wave, among swimming bacteria you can often see a sort of conductor, showing the rest of them how to swim.

To observe the awesome reproductive capacity of a bacterium, which in a colony's explosive growth phase can divide every twenty minutes (so that in three hours there are over a thousand from that single one and in fifty hours there would theoretically be 10^{45} bacteria, a volume larger than the earth itself), produces almost the same impression as watching the performance of a Gypsy Moth or an ant queen-mother. It reminds us that germs and insects are wherever we go; that there are ten million, maybe up to thirty million, species of insects, more than any other class or taxa of the visible animal world; that the insects, just like microbes, penetrate the biosphere dozens to thousands of metres deep and kilometres high in the atmosphere; that the biomass of insects on the planet is bigger than the biomass of all the other creatures put together; and that if the nuclear winter set in, the insects would remain as the highest form of life.

With insects, as with germs, we can be certain of one thing: we have not yet described a sizeable percentage of the existing species, and probably never will in some cases, for example in the Amazonian rain forests, where they may become extinct before we can penetrate their invisibility.

Insect colonies and microbe colonies have the common feature of integration in a single supraorganism or under-thought, in which individuals are totally expendable and easily replaceable units. We don't mind that where germs are concerned. We don't try to understand it or feel it. But it shocks us in insects, even though as individuals they share few characteristics with us, just something like a front end and a back end and feet down below.

The phenomena of an ant-hill can be much more realistically understood by watching pneumococci in necrotic lung tissue than from those cute little fellows in the comic strips and cartoons.

Incomprehensibility is more easily accepted in an invisible world, but that is what Bacon calls *idolum mentis*, an illusion of the mind. There is nothing more comprehensible about the Hercules beetle, the size of a skinny rat, than about a rickettsia. Although we can see the beetle, we know nothing, or very little, about the signals creating its image of the world.

The consequence of the apparent comprehensibility of the visible and the happy incomprehensibility of the invisible is simple. Germs can't surprise us by anything they do, whereas insects surprise and frighten us wherever we go.

A layman is not very surprised (and therefore not very frightened) that even though bacteriological medicine is in good shape, as opposed, say, to virological medicine, new diseases that result from bacterial infections continue to crop up — for example, Lyme disease (provoked by a relatively new type of Borrelia) or stomach inflammations related somehow to Campylobacterium pylori, or the notorious Legionnaires' disease, which led to the discovery of a new genus with seven species that existed both in ancient waters and in recent aerosols.

Run-of-the-mill bacteria (strains of Escherichia coli) complicate each other's lives in our intestines by means of colicins, which are toxic for other strains of the same species owing to receptors on their surfaces that mix them up with vitamins or iron carriers — yet these facts are not found particularly inspiring or breathtaking.

In the domain of the invisible, we do not find it surprising or positively frightening that we can put the gene for human insulin into E. coli, and by swapping a few amino acids create a mutation, so that insulin with better qualities of non-coagulation and stability is produced, insulin better than the insulin made by the good old pancreas. If we could do something like that with insects, it would trigger off a massive wave of anti-science fiction about flies with human heads and human thoughts, insulin notwithstanding.

Even a citizen whose apartment isn't overrun with pharaoh ants grins in amazement to learn that hormones analogous to their juvenile hormones have been developed and used by the

Prague chemistry school to suppress the metamorphosis of ant larvae into adults that might crawl around in the cupboard. Germs, on the other hand, don't seem to crawl anywhere, and chemotherapy, as far as he's concerned, is just a pill among other pills.

We learn about the lyrical and dreadful aspects of the struggle for life by meditating not on colicins but on fireflies. The males and females attract each other by perfectly timed flashes of their luminescent organs. The females of the genus Photuris, once fertilized, no longer respond to the signals of their males; instead they answer signals of the males from the smaller genus Photinus, seducing them into attempted sex that rapidly turns into death in the mandibles of the Photuris brand.

These rhythms may be close to those of my pulsating caterpillars, though of course *they* weren't trying to attract anyone or anything. They wanted only to resemble one large animal, and they did it in a surprising way and with surprising accuracy.

Maybe only real insects, large as life, can show us convincingly what a microbial infection can look like, an infection otherwise perceived by a citizen only through distress, a thermometer and the immoderate consumption of antibiotics.

In my case, a systemic infection by insects went this way: as a student, greatly drawn to the mysterious ways of insects, I kept caterpillars of the Goat Moth in caterpillar boxes in my little rented room. The caterpillars, which look disgusting and resemble huge, shiny bacteria the colour of a mucous membrane, gnawed away silently and legitimately at the proffered poplar wood. I counted three moults, and the caterpillars began to resemble elongated pigs. At night I thought I could hear them smacking their lips in their boxes. Then they vanished; either my calculation of the moults was wrong — there were supposed to be four — or theirs was. They had definitely entered a wandering phase and wandered away. And they left my mind the way staphylococci leave a sick person, after the infection and before the outbreak of inflammation.

Then one day my dignified landlady turned up to take the carpet outside for a beating. She tried to roll it up and found she couldn't. It was fastened to the parquet by countless Goat Moth cocoons, each one inserted in a depression neatly nibbled out from the wood. The good woman fell into a fevered state; screaming deliriously, she stamped on the cocoons with her gigantic slippers, as they exploded greasily and juicily.

This was a case of hyperacute infection in an apartment accompanied by massive central symptoms in the landlady. I tried to call her attention to the interesting processes of tissue reconstruction in the cocoons and the interesting parallel to microbial mysteries. I don't think she appreciated these intellectual aspects of the situation. In a very short time I moved to another lodging.

The microbial nature of the insects' customs has stayed with me. Microbes cannot surprise us by anything they do. And insects surprise and frighten us wherever we go.

Growing Up

Carl Friedrich von Weizsäcker said that man is an experiment which cannot be interrupted halfway. Once begun, you have to finish it. If we agree that we are not at the end of the experiment but at the beginning, at the age when a child learns to live with others collectively, and if we agree that the formulation of questions and systematic answers belong to the experiment called man, then we can hardly do without science. Science has proved to be the most successful way to ask questions and find answers, one that cannot be replaced. If man is unthinkable without questions, man is unthinkable without science.

There is, however, a discrepancy between our general pre-adolescent mentality (demonstrated in our arts, according to Medawar) and the relatively adult way of asking questions in science. If we agree that we are destined to grow up instead of merely lingering in a state of immaturity, romantic – some-times hysterical (when facing death and other accidents) – we have to learn to live with organized science and its ways of thinking.

I am not saying it is 'better' to grow up and to ask grown-up, that is 'learned', context-dictated, unspontaneous questions. (Maybe it is not even better to learn words, algebra and good manners.) It is simply inevitable. And I have yet to hear protests against the driving licence, even though traffic laws represent serious restrictions on children's ideas and freedoms.

Growing up in the age of science is, however, complicated —
by concealed collective anger, by vain attempts to resuscitate
old myths and superstitions, and by the use of science as a
scapegoat for all the troubles caused by an imperfect civili-
zation and an imperfect social order. Meanwhile, the practical
consequences of research, such as advanced technology and
information systems (by which humanitarian ideals and non-
ideals are spread), are taken for granted.

The matter is further complicated because the relative
adulthood of science has had no immediate impact on the
biology of the scientists themselves. I think it was the insolent
Pitigrilli who said that only a ladies' ballet school could create
a situation worse than that in a research institute. This is not a
rule, but it is not unknown.

Yet what is essential about science as the first truly collective
planetary human enterprise is its relative independence from
the social, economic and political climate. It creates an
efficient and impartial system of correction and verification.
This system excludes gross contamination and interference
from both the inside and the outside. Only the final product of
research is submitted for judgement and projection; at this
point, brains from the other spheres of culture must partici-
pate, assuming they are real brains and not mere agglomer-
ations of superstition.

I can't see many reasons for a poet claiming expertise in
palaeolithic cave paintings or the psychology of Cro-Magnon
man on the one hand, while ignoring the scanning electron
microscope and the psychology of a surgical team on the other.
To believe 'nature' is closer to the palaeolithic era than to the
surgery of pain is misleading; to believe that for the palaeo-
lithic era we do not need decades of expert, that is scientific,
erudition is fatal. The rejection of science is often the rejection

of tiresome reading and strenuous thinking – which the more or less privileged poetic mind tries to replace with insights and feelings, brief communications and lines of least resistance. I do not doubt the privileged status of some – few – poetic minds, but we should never confuse laziness with the privileged status.

The educational pressure created by science is serviced by schools and by the mass media. I believe that it is natural to proceed from the small certainties and basic data of contemporary science, communicated at school, to the great uncertainties and conceptions, as elegant as they are transitory, which should be communicated by the popularizing media. The main problem of scientific popularization is that it is controlled by the popular, urgent (and often justified) questions of laymen, instead of by what science can really solve.

Popularization that restricts its agenda to the reproduction of all *a priori* popular questions and false promises – frequently formulated by researchers craving fame – is, at best, a diversion, like a pub selling scientific draught beer. Popularization should be accessible – but not at any cost. And the degree of comprehensibility should be at the level not of the passive and idle consumer, but of a reader able to appreciate the pleasure of complications and obstacles which have been overcome.

In many fields, the beauty of a thought or experimental operation is impossible to communicate in popular ways, yet at least some approximate generalizations can be endowed with the beauty of elegant and imaginative language. In this sense, real popularization requires the same talent as a real poem. It should not become the domain of writers who simply cannot do anything else. The best form of writing about science is the essay, by Lewis Thomas, say, which presents selected problems and the scientific way of thinking in a refined literary form.

To learn how to co-exist with the system of organized science and its thinking does not mean we are all going to understand each other completely, but it means that we will all know our limits.

After all, to know one's limits is one of the signs of growing up.

Transplantation as a Literary Lapse

Some time ago I was asked to be the special adviser on a Czech crime film. The main plot depicted the following incident: the villain, wishing to steal the brilliant invention of a Czech scientist, gropes for the relevant papers in a safe where test tubes with a culture of tetanus bacilli are also stored. The villain cuts his finger on a test tube and is subsequently exposed when he exhibits symptoms of the disease. I thought my main advisory duty was to get rid of this plot, because medical documents would probably be stored together with tetanus cultures only during earthquakes of 8 to 9 points on the Richter scale, and test tubes would be put in a safe only during a fire affecting all laboratory equipment. Besides, I insisted, you could break a test tube while reaching into a safe only by performing a karate chop and hitting the test-tube stand, an action seldom executed by villains creeping around in the dead of night.

But advice of this sort was absolutely unwelcome. I was kindly told that my job was to show how to give a guinea pig a shot, and what tetanus should look like on the surface of a villain, but I was not to criticize the fundamental ideas, because they enjoyed artistic licence.

Abashed, and on the advice of more experienced advisers, I then advised actor Jan Pivec how to reach into a safe, where a tetanus culture had been accidentally placed, accidentally in a cracked test tube, accidentally on the research papers of an accidentally brilliant inventor. I must say Mr Pivec was perfect as the villain in the guise of a kind-hearted goody; he demonstrated despair and tetanus as if he had suffered from clostridial infections since childhood. The artistic licence was thus even more prominent.

No objections to licence, of course; but why should it apply only to the plot and not to secondary circumstances? Why should injections be administered just as they are in reality, and why should a laboratory look like a laboratory and not like Doctor Caligari's cabinet, which would have been more appropriate in view of the plot? Particularly where science is concerned, one would like consistency. In art, such consistency is also called style. But on the whole a minor lapse in plausibility is no big deal, as we all know.

It is worse when lapses in plausibility, consistency and professionality are deliberate. For instance, the artist, let us say a writer, decides that those poor researchers lack imagination, or lack some really ethical and deeply human insight, and he will remedy this shortcoming in his work of art. Then, because the audience, including artists, has had many more personal experiences with doctors than, for example, with palaeontologists, the remedy will usually involve medical problems, not the study of stegocephali, even though stegocephali could be studied more easily than internal medicine. The author is irresistibly drawn to surgeons – mainly because their performance is more visible, photogenic and heroic than the deeds of someone like a gastroenterologist.

The further we are from professionalism, the easier it is to commit lapses in the name of imagination and deep human insight.

As far as I know, none of the great Czech physicians and scientists who were also writers, such as Vladislav Vančura,

Frantisek Langer, Antonin Trýb or Jaromír John, attempted to write science fiction or to tackle the ethics of the medical or other scientific disciplines, although they must have had some opinions about their professions — or original professions. Even a brief attempt shows that scientific imagination depends on mountains of literature and rivers of technology, and the first 'moral principle' is 'truthful thinking', suggested long since by Blaise Pascal. Even the first step of science (including biomedical science) into literature — that is, scientific essay writing — can be successfully and properly undertaken only by the top experts in a given field.

Otherwise, what emerges is a haphazard phantasmagoria which may be funny, but which science finds extremely repulsive, because it contradicts the original conception of science fiction — which is a certain extension of science into the future or into present life, as conceived by the best authors, rather than an extension of anti-scientific emotions into institutionalized science.

The remarkable shift from science fiction to anti-science fiction was made possible by the discovery that the second half of the term could be used against the first, that fiction could be slopped over scientific knowledge, even over real-life settings and situations, and that it could replace laborious studies of the scientific and technical backgrounds of subjects. Such fiction was and is an excuse for professional — I mean the literary profession's — laziness. What used apologetically to be called licence has turned into the present virtue made out of necessity, denoted science fiction.

Therefore, if we want to carry out a literary transplantation of the spinal cord in the conditions of a present-day district hospital, using totally contemporary characters (in these literary transplantations the relationships are greatly enhanced by including the problem of a live donor), and we meet with a protest from a consulting specialist, we can simply call the whole thing science fiction. The specialist can go where I went with the tetanus culture in the safe. Consistency and style – in the author's conception – have been saved; the adviser is a nitpicker.

Organ transplants, with or without the assistance of science fiction, supply ideal conditions for the preservation, by literature, of the purity of science. Live donors are particularly rewarding when doing consciousness transplants (just such a Hungarian novel has been translated into Czech, but neurophysiologists have not been impressed). If the donors are not alive, then the chosen subject is apt to be the problem of the clinical death of the donor and the supply of organs. Many literary and dramatic versions have one feature, one lapse, which is manifested as the meaning of the work: the essence of the pre-transplant situation is seen as a matter of individual interaction – waiting recipient who has not much time left, donor who has just been brought into the hospital, and surgeon who, torn by his responsibility to save this or that life, makes the fatal decision.

The whole human and medical process is thus reduced to the conflict in one mind, while ethical and other conclusions are drawn from it. The authors totally neglect – or ignore – the fact that a transplant involves extensive working teams and technical facilities, which may not form a philosophical, but undoubtedly constitute a factual basis for the decision-making process. No one makes or can make a personal choice for the donor and the recipient without having specific background materials submitted by others, other laboratories and other working teams, both near and very far. And by a computer, what is more. When thrashing out a basic 'philosophical' transplant situation, the authors completely leave out of account the existence and the distressed condition of masses of people on the waiting list.

This transplantation literature mirrors fundamental and widespread misunderstandings about the nature of medical and scientific work. The time of private researchers and hermits is long gone. These surgical performances are basically the work of a team, a function more of the discipline than of the individual state of one head and one pair of hands. Heads and hands, naturally, can be either better or worse, knowledgeable or less knowledgeable, but finally, from the beginning of erudition, they are deeply conditioned by both the narrow and the broader environments of specialization.

As to literature, one can recommend a sentence by Susan Sontag, one of the brightest theoreticians of contemporary art: 'The old conception of culture . . . defines art as criticism of life . . . The new sensibility understands art as an extension of life – meaning a reflection of new registers of life intensity.'

Or, to be blunt, one can recommend a sentence from the prayer of a seventeenth-century English nun: Protect me from the fatal habit of thinking I must say something on every subject and on every occasion . . .

If Kant Were Around Today

When, in the conclusion of his *Critique of Practical Reason*, Kant speaks of his famous starry heavens and moral law, he becomes for a moment a poet:

I see them confront me and link them immediately with the consciousness of my existence. The first [the wonder of the starred heaven] begins from the place I occupy in the external world of sense, and expands the connection in which I find myself into the incalculable vastness of worlds upon worlds, of systems within systems, over endless ages of their periodic motion, their beginnings and perpetuation. The second [the wonder of the moral law within] starts from my invisible self, from my personality, and depicts me as in a world possessing true infinitude which can be sensed only by the intellect. With this I recognize myself to be in a necessary and general connection, not just accidentally as appears to be the case with the external world. Through this recognition I also see myself linked with all visible worlds. The first view of a numberless quantity of worlds destroys my importance, so to speak, since I am an *animal-like being* who must return its matter from whence it came to the planet (a mere speck in the universe), after having been endowed with vital energy for a short time, one does not know how. The second view raises my value infinitely, as an *intelligence*, through my personality; for in this personality the moral law reveals a life independent of animality and even of the entire world of sense. This is true at least as far as one can infer from the purposeful determination of my existence according to this law. This [determination] is not restricted to the conditions and limits of this life, but radiates into the infinite (trans. Carl Friedrich).

Kant becomes a poet here not so much by his choice of words as by the power of his images. He was in fact more critical of his verbal capacities than many a professional poet. In his introduction to the second edition of the *Critique of Pure Reason*, he complains that he lacks the gift of lucid expression and ventures to hope that others will help explain his intentions.

I would say that Kant's dimensions and Kant's sense of the dimensions of humanity bypass the usual distinctions; typecast roles and criteria are rejected and man is everything rather than a doggedly specialized worker in one, or the other, or a third culture. And in no case are the dimensions determined by this or that particular century.

However, we spend a lot of time and energy in the world of smaller dimensions reiterating and reassuring each other that poetry no longer is — and never was — what Newton characterized it as: a type of ingenious nonsense. Newton represented universal science for Kant, so we add that science no longer is and probably never was a diabolical product of the unholy trinity of Newton, Locke and Francis Bacon, as William Blake felt in Kant's time. Nor was it something that diminishes beauty by its own growth, as Tennyson later thought.

Ever since, in the same smaller world, we have been struggling with, on the one hand, the late Enlightenment arrogance of obtuse workers from the less invigorating branches of science and, on the other hand, the universal humanistic conviction that 'science' and wisdom have been divorced in the last 200 years, and will perhaps continue to be for some years to come. Verlaine, *poète maudit* and bitter spirit of European poetry, regards science in his poem 'Wisdom' ('Sagesse') as the theft of forbidden fruit. It is supposed to be what a wise man must never know.

The followers of alternative modes of investigation and cognition can hardly invoke Kant to support their various historical projections of 'artistic sensibility'. According to the authoritative conclusion of Cassirer's study on Kant,

> critical philosophy . . . also strives from the empirical and sensory to the 'intelligible', and it finds its fulfillment and its true conclusion only in the intelligible as the idea of freedom. But the path to this goal leads 'through the Herculean labor of self-knowledge'. Accordingly, no 'flights of genius' and no appeal to any sort of intuitive flashes have any weight here, but strict conceptual demands and necessities rule; here no immediate feeling of evidence, psychological or mystical, decides, but methodically performed analysis and the 'transcendental deduction' of the basic forms of knowledge . . . Hence, to step into the infinite it suffices to penetrate the finite in all its aspects . . .

Nevertheless, one of the possible sources of the cultural split that has divided the world of science and the world of human wisdom was Kant himself: the idea has been proposed by authors I respect as much as Kant, the authors of the Brussels school, Prigogine and Stengers, in their work *Order Out of*

Chaos (1984). History is ironical, and the history of ideas doubly so.

According to Kant, our perceptions have causes, things-in-themselves, composing the *a priori* noumenal world, accessible not to experience but to pure intuition (*Anschauung*). This intuition has two forms, space and time, one for the external sense, the other for the internal sense. When both forms are taken in the Newtonian framework, they exclude, among other things, any geometry other than the Euclidean. Pure reason is capable of terminating the infinite chains of intellectual, let us say scientific, knowledge by unifying ideas (soul, world, God, freedom, immortality) projected inside us as moral consciousness relating us to the higher, transcendent order. Systematic knowledge of objects and experience cannot bring anything new, but mainly forms the basis for transcendental reflection.

In this system, Prigogine and Stengers believe, science is attacked not for its limitations but for its essence. It is subordinated to a rival form of knowledge, and the field of scientific activity is locked into itself and separated from the world of values, of ethics and of freedom. Thanks to Kant's authority, here is the main divide that has dominated European thought and seen the birth of lyrical philosophies of the Bergsonian type – from which it is only a short step, Prigogine believes, to free speculation and the reward of poetic gymnastics whose mode is 'they doubt, but I know'.

The point is not so much a mistake inherent in Kant's system, as it is his romantic and stretching shadow. The dichotomy conceived by Kant was produced by the state of the sciences in his time, mainly the physics of solid bodies and astronomy. (If every later philosophical system were equally supported by the findings of contemporary science, at least in its framework, C. P. Snow would have had nothing to complain about.) Perhaps humanists and philosophers must accept that their systems are just as temporary as scientific theories.

Kant's thinking, hardly comparable with what we ruminate about in our time off, was based on a science of closed systems and universal laws, while the principal trait of present-day science is open systems, permanently exchanging energy, information and matter. These open, fluctuating systems exist not only in biology and anthropology, but also in physics and cosmology, and their study includes observers not only as intellectually predisposed individuals, but also as interested and involved operational units. Study also surpasses the possibility of an individual intellect; it stops being the activity of one private mind and becomes a team effort of people and machines.

If Kant were around today, he could hardly think of refuting the diversity of possible scientific views and of seeking a unified system of *a priori* principles. He would be the first to realize the significance of singularities at all levels, especially the cosmic singularity of life. We do not even face an *a priori* nature, imprinting our language on it; we face artefacts of genetic engineering, computer prognoses and models, a physics of plasma, superconductivity, chemistry of plastics and astronomy of black holes and quasars, 'reality' of eleven-dimensional supergravity.

The criterion of scientific existence is not only intellect and apparatus, but also something like unflagging imagination and moral resistance to failure, along with a tolerance for growing and undiminishing uncertainty. If this seems like news to some people, they must confuse the publishing of scientific results with the life of science itself. That is an increasingly misleading error, equivalent, in a way, to a unilateral loss of the imagination, which is available to the artist and the humanist for everything and at all times.

In contemporary science, more than ever before, the imagination is trained in a very surprising way. It has to achieve record times by running in the deep sand of accumulated knowledge. It works in the midst of such friction that the creation of new poetic metaphors is often closer, smoother and sweeter for science than for a professional writer's imagination – unless of course the scientific mind has got stuck at the level of late Newtonian scepsis about the ingenious nonsense of poetry, and in aesthetic colour-blindness.

It is, however, particularly necessary and topical to point out that the 'intelligence' – which 'raises the value infinitely' of 'personality' where 'the moral law reveals a life independent of animality and even of the entire world of sense' – means that existence 'is not restricted to the conditions and limits of this life, but radiates into the infinite'. The everyday practice of today's sciences covers not only the Kantian hypothetical imperative (you must behave in this way to achieve that result), but something like a categorical imperative as well, even though science cannot accept the imperative's supposed transcendental nature and noumenal position. Considered metaphorically, the categorical imperative, in Bertrand Russell's definition, simply means that some actions are objectively necessary without consideration of the result.

Morality has become a rather immoral word today, and there is no doubt that the scientist (just like the poet) carries syndromes of acquired moral deficiency which he picked up somewhere outside, transmitted in some cases by books and newspapers. Nevertheless, even the moral part of Kant's world is an integral part of present-day theoretical and experimental sciences. In 1974, Bronowski was straightforward about it:

How do we get this knowledge? By behaving in a certain way; by adopting an ethic for science that makes knowledge possible. Therefore, the very activity of trying to refine and enhance knowledge – of discovering 'what is' – imposes on us certain norms of conduct. The prime condition for its success is a scrupulous rectitude of behavior, based on a set of values like truth, trust, dignity, dissent, and so on. As I say in the book, 'In societies where these values did not exist, science has had to create them to make the practice of science possible.'

This fits in with the conception of the hypothetical imperative. The distressed researcher, who has amply learned his lesson from repeated failures and accidental successes, simply takes no risks and restricts himself to scrupulous behaviour and discipline, actions which would be a shining model in civil life. A sufficiently intelligent researcher dares not submit inauthentic results or adjust the obtained data, because especially in projects with a big impact he can never be sure that the undesirable discrepancy does not mean something. In all the cases of so-called scientific fraud in recent years, a stress situation was identified which affected the moral state of the hoaxer to such an extent that he stopped being himself.

But what about the technical assistant who is merely thanked at the end of the publication, is usually not personally or existentially interested in the results, has no scientific ambition, and only does his or her technical, ordinary, tedious job? The person puts himself or herself out by sticking to the rules, by admitting the everyday mistakes, and definitively by supplying results in which nine laboratory animals produce values of 90 to 120 and the tenth a value of 600, when you cannot really say the tenth one (technically known as the 'idiot-mouse') is different in any way.

This technical assistant, usually female, really exists in many a laboratory, and we are all dependent on this person, that is, dependent on the categorical imperative by which this person is ruled – nobody knows why. The point is not that this technical assistant is a nice and honest person; when the syndrome of acquired moral deficiency is spreading, these words become synonyms for simple-mindedness. The technical assistant does all these things without expecting that the value of his or her personality will be infinitely elevated and reveal existence radiating into infinity. As a rule, he or she cannot even expect the revelation of adequate financial compensation; the ridiculous emolument must be divided among a mathematical set of so-called technical assistants who develop maximum energy in order to do nothing.

Such a person is the personification of the categorical imperative in conditions difficult to imagine even for a head like Kant's. However, such a person is the *sine. qua non* of present-day science.

There are, of course, situations in basic research when actions occur between the involved scientific parties that are 'objectively necessary without consideration of the result'. Even carefully checked and repeated experiments occasionally produce results that contradict the fundamental laws on which present-day science is based. This happened recently with the results of an international team which had observed antibody activity in dilutions so extreme that they absolutely excluded the presence of antibody molecules as such. The only explanation was something fantastic – a configuration of water molecules mirroring a configuration of formerly present molecules of protein. The study was published in the renowned magazine *Nature*, although it disputed solid evidence of 200 years and supplied arguments for anti-scientific speculations. It was neither in the interest of the magazine, nor in the interest of immunochemistry, and maybe not even in the interest of the authors themselves to have the study published. But it was published, with an editorial comment written under the evident categorical imperative that unless there is a proof that information is disinformation, it must not be suppressed.

In the not yet fully appreciated history of Czech biology and medicine in the early 1950s, researchers can be found who could not be taught, even by loss of employment, to close their eyes to laboratory, clinical and agricultural experiments that contradicted the orthodox scientific criteria and standards and went under the banner of dialectic materialism of Lysenko or even poor old Pavlov. At that time it was rather uncertain whether there would be science again. In other words, the categorical imperative was equal to the scientific conspiracy of silence – and science survived, here and there, in one man's head and at the base of another man's skull.

Basic research and its imperative turn up with increasing frequency in everyday practice, and they bring with them risks – indirectly proportional to the moral principles that have followed the work from its inception. Social practice, a euphemistic expression for global risks, multiplies the human factor and makes it dramatically visible. In large-scale technologies, laboratory mice become riders of the Apocalypse, ticking atomic clocks are planetary bells. Under the powerful magnifying glass of big technologies the moral qualities of the entire human process are drastically revealed, from the idea to the factory.

It is generally known that the Chernobyl tragedy was not caused by failures of physics and technology, but by chronic failure in people. According to Yuri Scherbak's testimony, V. A. Legasov (a physicist studying nuclear technology, the chemical problems of plasma and the synthesis of compounds of rare gases), who came to clean up the disaster in 1986, said:

> In the past, in the thirties and forties, people creating technology were educated in the spirit of principles of supreme humanism. That kind of education was built on outstanding literature. On real art. On beautiful and correct ethical principles . . . This moral imperative was the basis of everything — relationships among people, relationship to humanity as such, relationship to technology and one's duties . . . Human morality was given its due in modern technology . . . But in the following generations . . . many engineers grew up from a utilitarian, technocratic foundation, and they saw only the technical side of the matter. If someone is weaned on technical ideas, he can merely multiply technology, or perfect it at best, but nothing principally new can be expected from him. The low level of expertise and insufficient sense of responsibility of the people [who caused the Chernobyl disaster] is not the cause but the consequence. The consequence of their lacking ethical qualities.

Today, technology must be protected from man, said Legasov. He meant from men who lack the imperative of precision and perfection in their performance — the imperative connected by some loose end to the moral imperative, no matter from whom it was caught.

If Kant were around today, I say he would devote himself to negative entropy, hypotheses about the origin of order in chaos, and theories about the spontaneous growth of complexity in closed stationary systems with a constant flow of energy, just like Prigogine; and just like Prigogine, he would hate free speculations and would still hold on to the categorical imperative on all levels. At least in the sense of the statement uttered by Uncle Gottfried in Romain Rolland's *Jean Christophe*: 'Do what you can, the others don't even do that!'

On Kindness

A long time ago I was tested in the field of biochemistry. It wasn't then a science very dear to me. Now, everyone knows there are times in human ontogeny when the heart is wholly opposed to biochemistry, except for some hormone receptors, and at the time I wasn't very sure about proteins or sugars, or even fats. Professor Hamsík, who was tall, bony and kind, finally asked me an unusually simple question: 'Where, in which system of the body, are antibodies manufactured?' He wanted me to say, 'In the reticuloendothelial system,' but let's skip over that terrible word; it isn't true any more anyway, at least not completely. But I, ruined by some preceding rigorous question, answered reflexively, 'In the urogenital system, Professor.'

It was a stupid answer. The Professor, however, nodded his head understandingly and said, 'Yes, certainly, dear colleague, but with the qualification that this system would be somewhat . . . um . . . penetrated by the cells of the . . . well?' I stammered: 'The nervous system, in light of the teachings of Pavlov.' But Professor Hamsík, evidently concerned that I could not connect even the pituitary gland to all of this, said, 'You wanted to say reticuloendothelial system, didn't you, but somehow it slipped your mind, isn't that it? Is a B-minus good enough?'

It was good enough. It wasn't. But I thanked him sincerely, and a certain glow spread between us – the glow of kindness.

It's the glow in which B-minuses are a great victory of the spirit, in which all systems are the same, and in which the truth comes out anyway since a person can't resist looking up the correct answer afterwards, and doesn't forget it for the rest of his life. And what's more, the production of antibodies became my life's work: I'm now an immunologist in a Prague research institute.

And if now and then I find some quality missing in myself or in the people around me, it hasn't anything to do with antibodies, but with the glow of kindness.

After all, as the cards have fallen, the important thing in life hasn't been to give the correct answer when I'm on the spot OR ELSE, but to have felt a warm and strong hand give me a nudge — just a little one — that helped get me out of some dark corner I'd got myself into.

You see, pounding a fist on a desk is easy, but the correct answers are easy too, when you think about it. At the very least they can be learned. But not kindness. Kindness just has to exist, perhaps coming from some great merit, from great suffering, or from some great intention. And only through kindness do exams in biochemistry, like life itself, become memorable.

Maxwell's Demon or, On Creativity

When hearing or saying the word 'creativity', one is supposed to put on a dignified, even pious expression – but modest as well, as if it did not concern us. Of course, every member of the so-called creative professions thinks it concerns him very much, and by the size of his modesty he artfully implies the supposed size of his divine spark. The modest look is appropriate, since the divine spark is usually related to touches of human craziness, and not even a quite extensive detour can avoid them. It should not be forgotten that the criteria accepted for the evaluation of the products of creativity – uniqueness, novelty, the element of surprise, elegance of solution – are conditions met to a remarkable extent by the paintings of schizophrenics. I used to own a whole gallery, the value of which became apparent after their loss during a move to another place. I can say I used to put on a very modest face, even deep inside, when looking at them – and I would have never allowed any claims for my own creativity. I was enacting a popular saying quoted by P. B. Medawar: I may not be absolutely brilliant, but at least I am not out of my mind.

Somehow, Plato's divine rapture of creativity, Pascal's sentence '*l'extrême esprit est voisin de l'extrême folie*,' and Lombroso's almost clinical correlation of genius and psychic deviation still linger in our minds. Creativity remains surrounded by a mist or aureole, copiously fed by the Romantic literary tradition and the seemingly scientific soul-searching

Freudian and post-Freudian conceptions. Creativity still has more to do with Wordsworth's 'sense sublime', 'Whose dwelling is the light of setting suns . . . and in the mind of man', than with the anthropic principle in the universe, more to do with the superego than with unified field theory or the notion of the selfish gene. One of the reasons for this is that operating with archetypes and myths is more conspicuous and rewarding. Over a hundred years ago, Matthew Arnold wrote that 'the critical power is of lower rank than the creative', and many people still hold to that opinion, even though the idea is not much canvassed any more. As late as 1960, however, Harold Taylor stated that 'the subconscious has a new status and often gets mixed up with creative imagination.' Generally speaking, every idea with some poetic value appears more creative than an idea reduced to its components, verified and sieved, criticized and revised by scientific creation.

It is understandable, in an epoch of expansive growth of science and technology – their material effects and sometimes even conceptual penetration into the life of men – that the soul of art should look for its refuges and inalienable domains. When the other schoolchildren rode bicycles and some were even driven in their parents' cars, I ascribed (in my mind) considerable moral and existential qualities to my scooter, and I would have liked to adorn it with symbolic wings, had I known how. I definitely thought riding a scooter was much more creative. The concealed argument of art turns on creativity – either as firebird, or as shrinking violet. Not entirely candidly, this argument is pitted against the apparently mechanical large-scale entrepreneurship of science.

There is not only this syndrome of withdrawal to unassailably higher ground. Man's creativity is mainly visible in man himself. 'Man is the first and principal self-creating creature,' wrote Lewis Mumford, to which the anthropologist Loren Eiseley added:

> And art plays an enormous role in the act of self-creation. It is art that touches the hidden chords of compassion, searches in our heart, makes us sensitive to beauty, asks about determination and destiny. Although these questions always lurk behind all the corners of the external Universe, which is the privileged domain of science, the strictness of scientific method does not allow us to follow them directly.

In this sense, creativity in art is immediately visible and significant because it is necessarily homocentric, and is part of a tradition (since art is a permanent self-reflection not only of man but also of its own ways). Moreover, the voice of the artistic creative act does not vanish in the not-so-resounding field of atoms, molecules, cells and stars.

Also, it is easier to cite creativity as the source of a highly personal and unique artistic performance than to propose it for cumulative, communal, transferable and, to some extent, replaceable scientific product.

Scientific creativity might be distinguished by the combination of imagination with critical and technical judgement, or at least by not putting the two in factual contradiction. Synergy between imagination and strictly rational reflection conditioned by extensive knowledge of literature, synergy between free invention and consistent immediate criticism, is regarded by P. B. Medawar as 'the greatest of all discoveries' – in the understanding of this synergy may lie the key to the conception of scientific creativity.

Contemporary psychological tests of creativity are based on hundreds of criteria, which at first sight do not arouse any suspicion that scientific creativity is being discriminated against in favour of artistic creativity. In general usage, however, creativity is still felt to be a breezy and blowing thing, the source of immediate snappy connections, and a machine with an exclusively 'artistic' emotional drive. In fact, I have never noticed that emotional drives are negligible in scientific creativity. The contrary is true. On the other hand, it was T. S. Eliot and no other who wrote in 1919: 'Poetry is not a turning loose of emotion, but an escape from emotion; it is not the expression of personality, but an escape from personality. But, of course, only those who have personality and emotions know what it means to want to escape from these things.'

If creativity is defined as an elegant or cute or appealing solution, whereas the truthful solution applies only to intelligence (Jackson and Messick, 1965), then it is easy to understand why Aristotle's conclusion that women have fewer teeth than men (in spite of the fact that he was twice married) is remembered more frequently among creative artists than his scientific observation that the spotted hyena is not a hermaphrodite.

Creativity tinged with that romanticizing hue naturally does not appear to be an indisputably positive feature in situations requiring rigid, consistent and unchanging intellectual control. Beware of creative surgeons, I was recently told by a psychiatrist friend.

As a matter of fact, psychiatrists need this creativity much more than surgeons, and this prompts a question: to what extent can creativity substitute for technology? To what extent can creativity – for instance in a laboratory or a workshop – become a remedy for material poverty, a sort of 'virtue out of necessity'? Probably to a very negligible extent. The final effect of 'virtue out of necessity' is more of the moral than material sort, and creativity often becomes the sister of futility. A patient will not be very enthusiastic about his healer's creativity if he does not receive the best possible medicine. Utilitarian questions such as 'Under what circumstances?', 'For what purposes?' and 'For what benefit?' cannot satisfactorily be cut off from the notion of creativity.

Historically, all this is undoubtedly simpler: the role of a writer, or even great writer, great painter, discoverer of penicillin or electromagnetism is directly embodied in a time-tested creative performance which was unique, new, surprising, elegant. Now, at a time of collectivization and institutionalization of scientific or even artistic creativity – when you can be a researcher without major results, sometimes even without doing much research, and an artist without an excess of divine rapture – roles are assigned by context and not necessarily because of some actual performance. Creativity is, introspectively at least, an automatic attribute of the role; creativity becomes a sort of automatic qualification, like graduating from a course or taking an eyesight test.

It follows from this that neither in art nor in science can one speak of creativity where simply learning a necessary technique and productivity is concerned, either out of tradition or through some other kind of inertia. While creativity usually presupposes erudition, it is not replaceable by erudition. Production of stereotypes, no matter how beautiful and successful they may be, is not a demonstration of creativity. It can be only a reminiscence of it, because creativity as a quality has its ontogenesis, its stages of flourishing and significance, and its stages of decline or insignificance, frequently compensated for by experience.

The first artefact of its kind can be the result of creativity, but not the second. The first elegant solution is creative, not a second similar one. Creativity, in the true sense of the word, cannot be a mere source of perpetual activity on one level, but must be the source of permanent change, a source of acquisition, a stimulus to proceed to a new stage, a cause of new waves on the broad surface of culture – new, unique, surprising, elegant waves.

From this the inference is that activity forced by creativity is no doubt hectic and manic, requiring bigger sources of energy than usual and greater resistance to trouble than usual; because even small-time Prometheuses have their small-time eagles, sometimes called flies. For the outstanding Czech literary critic F. X. Šalda, a 'genuine poetic work is the result of human creativity; and creativity is mainly found where there is a higher vitality than elsewhere'.

Creativity in art materializes in a specific performance, in a work proportional to creativity, whereas creativity in science (comprising the imaginative, critical and technical stages) often merely opens a problem space which consequently has to be filled with years of routine, collective and not very visible effort. It is clear, therefore, how much easier and more topical is the assessment of creativity undertaken by artistic criticism than the process of collective verification which represents scientific criticism. The less manifest scientific creativity is at the time, the less arguable its assessment when looking back. I would even say its results bring more satisfaction and it is less timid. And maybe scientific creativity is needed more in synthetic discoveries which open new territories than in analytical discoveries which map out territories already known.

In his *Two Cultures*, C. P. Snow fully recognizes how right Rutherford was, when to the remark 'What a lucky man, this Rutherford, still riding on the crest of the wave,' he replied:

'Yes, but it was I who made that wave.' Which must be the bluntest statement about creativity I know.

Among other things, it comprehends the simple and pure contradiction between creating and creation, a contradiction not to everyone's liking. Waves are made in water or another environment producing vibrations. They cannot be made from nothing. Creating does not make something out of nothing, but it introduces new kinetics into an already present environment – new organization of an already given space.

It reminds me of the paradox of Maxwell's demon and its solution. Just like creation and creating, the demon defied the second law of thermodynamics and recalled the famous Schrödinger metaphor about the essence of life being the suction of negative entropy from the environment. Maxwell's demon is something like an operational metaphor, a part of the functional poetry of modern science. It is a tiny fictitious creature, infinitely more capable than we are with our statistical laws; a creature changing disorder into order and non-usable energy into usable energy – a creative creature. It looks after a small sliding door which moves without friction between two separated compartments of a container filled with gas, that is, filled with whirling molecules of gas, no matter what they look like in our imagination. When a fast-moving molecule of gas comes from the left, the demon half-opens the door; when a slow molecule approaches, he keeps the door shut. If the demon keeps doing this long enough, without getting tired, all the fast molecules accumulate in the right-hand compartment, while the slow ones remain in the left one. There will be hot gas on the right, cold gas on the left. Or the demon will let in all the molecules from the right and none from the left, so eventually there will be a surplus of molecules from the left or all of them, and a shortage or nothing on the right. There will be order and difference in concentration, a possible source of energy. In terms of energy, Maxwell's creature of genius created something out of nothing by the mere act of molecular selection.

Alas, Maxwell's demon was banished, after haunting physics for years, by Leon Brillouin and his application of information theory. According to Harold Morowitz, Brillouin argued that the demon would have to base his performance of opening the door on observation, that is, on taking measurements in his environment. He would need photons or another physical signal to see the molecules. Any physical signal requires a release of energy. This release of energy brings about a proportional increase of entropy, which diminishes with the opening and closing of the door at the right moment. Not even information can be obtained out of a physical nothing.

So much for the demon.

I would also say that Maxwell's demon is a fit parable for the idea still evoked by the term 'creativity'. Does not such a demon sit by the cradle of every poem, and does it not let words through the door of the mind, heart and other metaphorical organs? Does it not separate fast words from slow words, does it not create order out of chaos and randomness? Higher energy from lower energy? Does it not create unforeseen and unprecedented information? Is it not the originator of creation – creation as the activity of a demiurge, not a mere carrier of energy? Does it not feed on negative cultural entropy?

Certainly, that is how we can imagine it. But the essential thing about the demon is that he does not exist.

Only the total intricacy and opacity of the human life cycle prevents – probably – analysis of the energies and dependencies of something that is sooner or later manifested as an act of creation and that apparently comes out of the blue. Of course, according to Maurice Merleau-Ponty, 'a gesture of the body towards the world brings the body into an order of relationships that mere psychology or biology knows nothing about', but Maxwell's demon was also abolished not only by the good old physics and mechanics of solid bodies but by something completely new. Anyway, it is difficult to agree with Merleau-Ponty on the act of creation because it is hard to make a statement when his verbal avalanches drop on your head: as Medawar remarked, you are in a state of 'reverential attention' before this 'prancing, high-stepping quality, full of self-importance; elevated indeed, but in the balletic manner, and stopping from time to time in studied attitudes, as if awaiting an outburst of applause. It has had a deplorable influence on the quality of modern thought in philosophy and in the behavioural and "human" sciences.'

In other words, one must decide whether to be uplifted by one's conception of creation or whether to try to understand it; whether to be enchanted with oneself or to try to learn about oneself.

It really does not matter whether we say and see a hand, a painting, a pen, tenderness, a memory, a face, sadness, morning, a smile, death, hope, a rose, night, eyes, on the one hand, or 10^{10} bits of genetic information, 10^{13} bits of nerve information and 10^{16} bits of human 'extrasomatic' (cultural) information on the other – except that the former sounds much better. What matters is that the input into this concentrated fabric of connections called the soul is about as powerful as the output, so that the creative act is something like Hegel's 'transformation of the necessary into the accidental and vice versa', or Malraux's 'coherent deformation to which we subject the data of the world till we obtain the meaning'. Or, recalling Šalda's words above, it is a higher form of vitality in the first place: those who have steam need no demons.

I almost forgot – I like demons very much, just as I like black princesses and white dwarves. I just do not see why we should use the poor demons to understand the world or worlds more easily, or to improve the job references of creative professionals.

To strike a personal note, I must state that I have never felt anything like creativity and, even if I had, I would not be caught dead admitting it.

For me, 'creativity' is too luxurious a word, too richly coloured. What I know is the will for new things and the enjoyment of new things, and these are identical in science and art. I think scientific and artistic activities do not exclude one another, no matter how different their techniques are. It is all about energy or steam, all about transformations of energy.

The term 'creative profession' is totally unsuitable because it is conservative and discriminating, and does not capture the basic feature of permanent change and permanent growth by which creativity is determined.

Windmills

Highway 5 to San Francisco picks its way through the huge agricultural areas of the San Joaquin Valley and rises up to bare grassy hills visited by the wind from the sea. As we go on, an enormous three-tipped star emerges from behind the hill, a windmill composed of three elegant aluminium blades on a mast. Five windmills, one hundred windmills, vast fields of windmills. Some stand still, others turn in a light–heavy motion, one faster, the other more slowly, none of them so fast that the blades merge; all the stars seems to walk through the air with the inaudible energy of angels. As one company disappears behind a hill, another battalion of windmills emerges, and they are so tall and graceful that Don Quixote could hardly raise an objection to them.

And on the other side comes an echelon of monumentally tender aluminium bowling pins, like the right and left contours of a viola, but more parabolical; at random, following their own reflection, their own choice of breezes, they spin in a dreamlike and slightly spellbinding girlish motion, which would make even Sancho Panza hesitate.

And nothing else around, just the bare green hilltops and steely sky. The windmills are not related to anything, they are windmills in themselves with their wind, they are the only motion in the landscape along the highway, a perpetual, let us say eternal, motion.

These windmills produce power and they belong to things

called wind farms. There must be around ten thousand such windmills in California at the moment, built by small associations of enterprising people who receive sufficient tax relief to sell the generated electricity to the power network or to nearby organizations for the same price paid for power from old sources.

This is optimistically effective and effectively daring. To raise the wind must be very different from raising cows in small muddy lots among the foothills, in corrals where thousands of heads of cattle are squeezed in so as not to run too much, so as to gain weight. To raise the wind is a fleeting and abstract enterprise. To raise the wind is invisible. And beautiful, if you think of it.

I would say it is a kind of new beauty, the beauty of an artefact that may not be outside the arts, but is certainly outside the domain of museums. Taking into account what it looks like, what it is and what it means, it must be the best kind of artefact in this world of deserts, fertile fields, muddy enclosures and museums with alarm systems.

Yes, as far as fine art goes, I can hear some venerable old man of any era proclaiming that a bare hill and a condor gliding in the air are much more essentially beautiful than a bare hill with a walking windmill. That is possible, but the first example of scenery excluded the venerable man's own silhouette, while the other one accepts it.

Enjoying these peaceful feelings we continue on our way, speeding in the appropriate and customary fashion. The colourful super-saurian trucks thrust their way through from right and left; since they can advise one another on the radio about the position of radars and the movements of police patrols, they speed in a much more professional way. When more of them turn up, it is like driving in an avalanche. The air pressure shakes you uncontrollably and without any organic pity; 900 miles a day is an inorganic task.

But as the red–yellow driver's cabin passes you up there on the right, a hand with a puppet suddenly sticks out of the window. The puppet, a cross between Punch, a beaver and Piglet, bows respectfully and beckons with a paw. It keeps looking at you until it vanishes in the waves of traffic. There is nothing mocking about this puppet. It is definitely a positive type of puppet.

This Punch–Piglet – for which we should be nothing but an obstacle en route to the heart of the golden West by our mere existence in this traffic lane – takes the trouble to beckon to us in this inorganic motion of inertial matters. Punch–Piglet finds that we are people, too, and not windy cattle; Punch–P has fun by doing funny things for others, although it can hardly get anything out of it.

I am sorry, but my understanding of beauty (I would never use such a dreadful word in another connection) oscillates between these windmills and this Punch–Piglet.

Poetry and Science
The Science of Poetry/The Poetry of Science

The Greek poet Constantine Cavafy is best known for his poem 'Waiting for the Barbarians'. The poem in Queen's English goes like this:

What are we waiting for, gathered in the market-place?

The barbarians are to arrive today.

Why so little activity in the Senate?
Why do the senators sit without legislating?

Because the barbarians will arrive today.
Why should the senators bother with laws now?
The barbarians, when they come, will do the
 law-making.

Why has our emperor risen so early,
and why does he sit at the largest gate of the city
on the throne, in state, wearing the crown?

Because the barbarians will arrive today . . .

And so on. The consul and the praetors walk out in their scarlet, embroidered togas, wearing bracelets with sparkling emeralds and precious staves inlaid with silver and gold . . . because the barbarians will arrive today – and such things dazzle barbarians. Orators don't give their speeches . . . because barbarians are bored by eloquence . . . The poem concludes:

What does this sudden uneasiness mean,
and this confusion? (How grave the faces have become!)
Why are the streets and squares rapidly emptying,
and why is everyone going back home so lost in thought?

Because it is night and the barbarians have not come.
And some men have arrived from the frontiers
and they say that there are no barbarians any longer.

And now, what will become of us without barbarians?
These people were a kind of solution.

Listening to so many literary orators, senators and praetors, I have the recurring feeling that they really do believe in barbarians, in law-making barbarians, in barbarians bored by eloquence, even in barbarians threatening the sublime cultural edifices; barbarians who would be whole-hearted opponents of the artist's creative complex, of the preservation of the only and truly human nature protected by the arts and humanities; barbarians who would be at the same time a kind of solution to the inborn problems of ageing societies and cultures; who would at least provide an easy, silent target for traditional humanitarian emotions, passions and conservational tendencies.

The barbarians are of course the scientists.

The romantic disjunction of head and heart is, after 200 years, still not cured in an individual artist's mentality. The artist's primal and direct communication with the nature of man and things is still seen as an alternative and more genuine path of human creativity, opposing the analytical, cold and cynical scientific approach.

Science is spectrum analysis: art is photosynthesis, as Karl Kraus has put it. Or, according to the Polish satirist Stanislaw

Jerzy Lec, the hay smells different to the lovers than to the horses.

Let's take a look at the realm of the horses. Has it still the same constitution and structure it had during the Enlightenment and the Romantic reaction to the Enlightenment? Is the scientific paradigm, that is, the apparatus of perception and the framework into which all observations are fitted, unchanged throughout the last couple of centuries? Or are we confronted with a different paradigm from that which confronted the Encyclopaedists, the Rousseauians and the Herderians?

If there is something like a 'Science', that is a complex of activities creating methods for acquiring applicable information on the world, then it is not a perennial coral reef increasing by simple accretion, but a slow, frequently unnoticed transition from the First to the Second and Third Science.

In the First Science, introduced by the Ancient Greeks, the method consisted of forming axioms from which certain theorems could be deduced by the application of logical systems which would today be regarded as 'philosophical' rather than 'scientific'. In the Renaissance, the First Science was gradually replaced by the Second. This was based on systematized observation with the naked eye or with tools developed at that time. It invented the interrogation of nature through experiments, which in turn were based on assumptions derived from direct observations, on entities conveyed by observation, on entities very similar or identical to the data of everyday sensual experience. The paradigm of the Second Science resulted in an enormous wealth of classifications, descriptions and notions of objects and elementary forces. The Second Science is metaphorically represented by the reality of scientific libraries bulging with wisdom, aspiring to contain the world *per se* and the world for man, by the tons of

Handbücher and *systemata naturae*, and by the reality of scientific laboratories where uninvolved observers ask their questions and manipulate disparate objects, dissect them and rearrange them in chains of facts and abstractions.

In the extensive mechanism of the Second Science even intensive personalities like Kelvin or Darwin bore the signs of closeness and finiteness of their fields, which resembled rather an official agenda than an abyss.

The Second Science has enriched the vocabulary by an enormous wealth of terms and denotations attributed to natural objects and technological processes. At least in this respect it had a marked positive effect on the literary mind which followed the Second Science in the demythicization-by-denomination process, abandoning the broad notions of just trees, just flowers or just crafts and going for concrete, specific terms. At least in the descriptive approach to objects and forces the literary mind (and culture in general) made use of the Second Science paradigm.

Nevertheless, the devitalized library and the cool, white, unimaginative laboratory – the supposed idea of the Second Science – still represent a counterpoint to what we think of as the individual Artistic Mind, deep, warm and increasingly sophisticated in its introspection.

Frequently we find that artists believe, at least in private, that they are fundamentally opposed to this science, to inimical science which is designed to endanger their minds, their aims and their ways of life, as well as the homeostasis of the planet. They still believe in 'the Vulture whose wings are dull realities', as did Edgar Allan Poe in 'the crude composition of my earliest boyhood' in 1829. They content themselves on the one hand with a subnormal understanding, of the present sciences in particular, and with a pretended general understanding of 'Science' on the other, albeit they mix up science, technology and the application of both – which is rather the consequence of the given social structure than the responsibility of sciences. Some like to understand what they believe in. Others like to believe in what they understand, says Lec. This private artistic attitude amounts to a total misunderstanding, to a kind of artistic dogmatism and, at the same time, to artistic messianism. In Lec's terms, 'Every stink that fights the fan thinks it is Don Quixote.'

'. . . human kind / Cannot bear very much reality . . .', said T. S. Eliot.

It is astonishing how little change has occurred in the realm of lovers – in the mood and ideology of the traditional culture during the last eighty years. Almost the same controversy on culture, education and science developed in 1882 between T. H. Huxley and Matthew Arnold and in 1959 between C. P. Snow and F. R. Leavis. In both cases the issue was the impact of science, technology and industry on human life and on human values. But it was really Arnold who clearly understood what the Encyclopaedists, the French Revolution and Hegel told the world, namely that Reason, Idea or Creative Imagination had become decisive in human destiny.

Art was for Arnold a criticism of life, and literature, a central cultural act, was itself criticism of culture. But culture represented for Arnold 'the best that has been thought and said in the world'. Consequently, the opposition of culture and science, in Snow's terms of traditional culture and scientific culture, appears to be an artificial one. The 1959 controversy is a confrontation not of two cultures but only of two autoreflections of the artistic and scientific establishments – of the artistic sensibility, and the paradigm and material consequences of the Second Science.

The controversy has hit a soil so fertile that Peter Medawar, after twenty years, protests that his essay 'Science and Literature' could be taken as 'yet another contribution to this idiotic debate'.

However, we firmly believe with Susan Sontag that modern art is rather an extension of life than a method of knowledge and evaluation – and therefore subject to the same dynamic changes as technology and science. Hence there is very little left to argue about.

However, in this century, the paradigm of the Second Science has been broken up and is vanishing bit by bit, together with the psychological type of the private scientist with a mind prepared for the chance coming mostly late in the night. A new paradigm is emerging, that of Goodall's Third Science struggling with the 'fluent' nature of things. The first step was the new development of physics where the material world was found to consist of entities basically different from anything we can experience by our senses. 'The world of billiard ball atoms existing at definite times in simple three-dimensional space dissolved into the esoteric notions of quantum mechanics and relativity, which to the unsophisticated seem most "unnatural"' (C. H. Waddington). The world of living things, consisting so far of a hierarchical order of organisms, organs, cells and functions, was dissolved into torrents of evolution, molecular interactions, realizations and errors, all regulated by somewhat unhuman forces of genome and selection, proceeding not simply from the 'lower' to the 'higher' organization, but rather from the principle of minimal information to assure the preservation of that information to the principle of maximal conciseness of information. A rather 'revolutionary idea' emerged 'that chance and indeterminacy are among the fundamental characteristics of reality' (L. Trilling).

Interest has moved towards the study of general properties of systems of information and organization. By this tendency science has enclosed many areas so far unexplored and so far regarded as being out of the scope of the hard-centred scientific approach. Paradoxes like Maxwell's demon and the mysterious neurophysiology of the human brain are within its reach. This approach reveals, too, that every scientific field touched by something like the Third Science is incomplete 'and most of them — whatever the record of accomplishments over the past two hundred years — are stll in the earliest stage of their starting point' (Lewis Thomas).

But, most important, the involvement of the observer in the observed holds true in general (although this notion is still under dispute among physicists). The famous Heisenberg sentence maintains: 'Even in science the object of research is no longer nature itself, but man's investigation of nature.'

The root of the matter is not in the matter itself, as I put it in a poem.

The situation is beautifully defined by J. Robert Oppenheimer:

We have a certain choice as to which traits of the atomic systems we wish to study and measure and which we let go; but we have not the option of doing them all. This situation, which we all recognize, sustained in [Niels] Bohr his long-held view of the human condition: that there are mutually exclusive ways of using our words, our minds, our souls, any of which is open to us, but which cannot be combined: ways as different, for example, as preparing to act and entering into a retrospective search for the reasons of action. This discovery has not, I think, penetrated into general cultural life. I wish it had; it is a good example of something that would be relevant, if only it could be understood . . .

Last but not least, the present scientific paradigm and the organization of modern science provide a precise and lasting world memory and link distant causes with distant effects. They offer an operational framework of memory which was missing in the life of societies and in the culture.

No one of good will can fail to perceive current scientific events and their eminent role in our intellectual life. Science today 'is the way of thinking much more than it is a body of knowledge' and 'if science is a topic of general interest and concern — if both delights and social consequences are discussed regularly and competently in schools, the press, and at the dinner table — we have greatly improved our prospects for learning how the world really is and improving both it and us,' says Carl Sagan with a grain of idealism. And Lewis Thomas, who is definitely less exuberant, states: 'We need science, more and better science, not for its technology, not for leisure, not even for health and longevity, but for the hope of wisdom which our kind of culture must acquire for its survival.'

In my essay 'Science in the Unity of Culture', I referred to science as an ally of the intellect of the ordinary citizen; an ally helping him to make order out of disorganization, out of chaos, regardless of what forms these take. From the citizen's viewpoint, what we may loosely call the 'intellectual functions' of science and art overlap to form a unity, with each conditioning and complementing the other. This, of course, does not imply that the citizen lives all the time in the atmosphere of scientific and artistic tides; it implies only that they are within his reach when he has a chance to gasp the breath of culture.

In particular scientific disciplines which have sometimes

very little in common, the barbarians may well have created disparate images of a colourless world, cold and mute, alien to any sensual evidence. But at the same time they have subjected mankind to the pressure or freedom of basic and definitive technological progress; they have provided the human mind not only with new and innovative ideas, but also with new means of apperception, insight and expression. They have also produced the worldwide system of communications and the worldwide feeling of human simultaneity, as well as producing isolated, particular scientific universes with little possibility of intercommunication and translation into a universal scientific language. The universal paradigms are present rather by implication than in an explicit form.

It was William Butler Yeats who observed in 'The Return of Ulysses': 'The more a poet rids his verses of heterogeneous knowledge and irrelevant analysis, and purifies his mind with elaborate art, the more does the little ritual of his verse resemble the great ritual of Nature, and become mysterious and inscrutable.'

So, it is not only in the science–art relationship that we suffer or believe we suffer from the lack of a common language. It is also in the art–common-sense relationship. It is also within the arts themselves. Bronowski states that there is a general lack of a broad and general language in our culture. But it may be suggested that this lack is merely accidental, momentary and superficial. We may lack a common language and common sensibility, but we should be increasingly aware that we do share a common silence.

At first glimpse one might suspect that literature would be closer to the sciences than other art forms, because sciences also use words and depend on syntax for expressing their findings and formulating ideas. They have created specialized vocabularies of their own, mainly for purposes of higher precision and to approach the ultimate aim of highly formalized monolytic expression, if not a new syntax. Such a syntax has already been created by mathematicians and theoretical physicists. Writers use the same tools as scientists (except for mathematicians). They perform on the same stage, but move in the opposite direction. The sciences and poetries do not share words, they polarize them.

The assumption that a poet using scientific words, scientific vocabulary, could produce writing which would be closer to science and its spirit, without being a scientist himself is — to paraphrase Waddington — like rendering Shakespeare in the language and philosophical framework of an evening newspaper. Scientists publishing verses in the back pages of their professional magazines certainly engage in funny, witty and graceful exercises, but are as far from poetry as poet laureates making verses on the front pages of literary magazines on the perennial merits of Poetry, verses worn out for decades or centuries. Even a gifted poet and a major scientist in one person, like the Nobel laureate for chemistry in 1981, R. Hoffman, cannot render the essence of his science in poems and writes rather about circumstances. There is no common language and there is no common network of relations and references. Actually, modern painting has in some ways come closer to the new scientific notions and paradigms, precisely because a painter's vocabulary, colours, shapes and dimensions are not congruent to the scientist's vocabulary. Their vocabularies are not mutually exclusive, but complementary.

Many present scientific disciplines are represented by their wording, or are embodied in the words, or are even seen as the thing said. Poetry is not the thing said, but a way of saying it (A. E. Housman).

For the sciences, words are an auxiliary tool. In the development of modern poetry words themselves turn into objects, sometimes *objets trouvés*. For William Carlos Williams 'The poem is made of things – on a field.' Thus the poem dwells in a new space and a new time and is due in Williams's example to a 'strange arithmetic or chemistry of art: " – to dissect away / the block and leave / a separate metal: / hydrogen / the flame, helium the / pregnant ash . . ."' To paraphrase Heisenberg, the object of poetic research is no longer nature itself, but man's use of words. Hence poetry moves ahead, paralleling the scientific paradigm in the realm of language, into areas less comprehensible for a reader accustomed to forming coherent mental pictures from the sequence of phrases, that is to say, accustomed to the commonplace or scientific use of words.

There may be an essential trait involved: the basis of any art, at least in a modern sense, is exactly that which cannot be recorded by this art's specific means, that which surpasses them. The basis of poetry is the unpronounceable, the basis of a picture is the unpaintable, the basis of music is the unplayable and the basis of a drama is hidden beyond the action. Perhaps art is based on the immanent inadequacy of its means, while science insists on the adequacy, or at least the temporary adequacy, of its means. Art is a binding inadequacy and therefore it is close to life. Science is a binding adequacy, limited by its time and space. Science has to say everything. Art which would say everything would be its own grave, as shown by pseudo-art, which always contains instructions for the consumer and formulates the final and obligatory commonplace notions.

In the use of words, poetry is the reverse of the sciences. Sciences bar all secondary factors associated with writing or speaking; they are based on a single logical meaning of the sentence or of the word. In poetry, very definite thoughts occur, but they are not and cannot be expressed by words stripped of secondary factors (graphic, phonetic) and especially by words chosen so as to bar all possibilities except one. On the contrary, poetry tries for as many possible meanings and interactions between words and thoughts as it can. This is not only for its inner freedom, but also for the sake of communication with readers, for their own freedom. The poet uses 'these words because the interests whose movement is the growth of the poem combine to bring them, just in this form, into consciousness as a means of ordering, controlling and consolidating the uttered experience of which they are themselves a main part' (I. A. Richards). The experience or, more broadly put, the tide of impulses 'sweeping through the mind, is the source and the sanction of the words' (I. A. Richards). For the reader, the words of the poem are meant to reproduce similar, analogous or parallel plays of feelings, thoughts and interests, putting him for a while into a similar, analogous or related inner situation, leading to his particular response. Why this should happen, says Richards, is the mystery of communication. Who knows how often it happens per book, per reading or per lifetime. Definitely not as frequently as we pretend.

With the increasing sophistication and matter-of-factness of its actual and potential readership, the essential poetic communication or triggering needs fewer words and more condensation in Pound's sense (*dichten* = *condensare*).

One of the functions of words in a poem is to make pseudo-statements in Richards's terms. The sole function of words in the scientific paper is to make statements which are not an end in themselves, but the matter of verification for future experimentation or for a present or presented theory. The 'truth' of poetic statements is acceptable or verifiable by some attitude, within the framework of the mood, style and reference of the poem. By reference I mean the relationship to a system of routine statements, to common sense and to the literary traditions and contexts. 'The poetic approach evidently limits the framework of possible consequences into which the pseudo-statement is taken. For the scientific approach this framework is unlimited. Any and every consequence is relevant' (I. A. Richards).

Interestingly, at least in my mind, which may be affected by my profession, some essential scientific notions, postulates, laws, some basic stones of the scientific syntax cannot be modified, cannot be transformed into pseudo-statements even when used in a poem. The poem too has to keep some bones of the scientific skeleton of the world. The point is illustrated in my prose poem 'Žito the Magician':

To amuse His Royal Majesty he will change water into wine. Frogs into footmen. Beetles into bailiffs. And make a minister out of a rat. He bows, and daisies grow from his finger-tips. And a talking bird sits on his shoulder.

There.

Think up something else, demands His Royal Majesty. Think up a black star. So he thinks up a black star. Think up dry water. So he thinks up dry water. Think up a river bound with straw-bands. So he does.

There.

Then along comes a student and asks: Think up sine alpha greater than one.

And Žito grows pale and sad: Terribly sorry. Sine is between plus one and minus one. Nothing you can do about that.

And he leaves the great royal empire, quietly weaves his way through the throng of courtiers, to his home in a nutshell.

So, in the use of words and statements, poetry and science move in different and almost opposite directions. But they do not aim, in my mind, for opposite ends. One of them is a humility that resists the onslaughts of powerful, prevailing imbecility, verbal or otherwise.

The aim of a scientific communication is to convey unequivocal information about one facet of a particular aspect of reality to the reader, and to the collective, anonymous thesaurus of scientific data. The aim of poetic communication is to introduce a related feeling or grasp of the one aspect of the human condition to the reader, or to the collective mind of cultural consciousness. As person-to-person messages, both kinds of communication involve a definite time of the full intellectual or intellectual–emotional presence. In addition, both are concerned with the establishment of a lasting memory, of intellectual or intellectual–emotional debris in the individual mind and in the collective mind of culture. And both the scientific and poetic communications are a function of condensation of meanings, of the net weight of meaning per word, of inner and immanent intensity. Opposed to other written communications, they are – at their best – concentrates, time-saving devices. I have been repeatedly intrigued by hearing from scientific colleagues that they do read poetry, because it is short, instantaneous and rewarding on the spot, just as a good scientific paper should be.

And the notion of the specific high inner intensity shared by the scientific and poetic communication leads me to suggest that there is another common trait: the goal of gravitational force of sudden revelation, discovery or statement with a predictive value. Here we are actually referring more to the very scientific action than to the communication, and at the same time to the act of writing rather than to the completed poem. But we must not forget that even the present form of scientific papers is based on a proven narrative structure of introduction, technical elaboration and almost instantaneous presentation of the findings where the graphic, numerical or condensed textual statements sometimes attain the value of a revealing metaphor.

In some sciences, which are still fully dependent on the traditional syntax, a conscious application of some sophisticated literary forms may occasionally occur. So a form of platonic dialogue between Prof. Soma (the name standing for the advocates of a somatic mutation theory) and Prof. Line (for germinal line theory) has been chosen by F. C. Osher and W. C. Neal for an impressive confrontation of the theories of generation of diversity (GOD) in immunological recognition. The article was published among 'normal' scientific communications in *Cellular Immunology* (17:552, 1975). I'd even suggest that in these sciences the aesthetic value of the literary communication still counts, and may become a noticeable quality. George Orwell may have been right when he remarked: 'Above the level of a railway guide, no book is quite free from aesthetic considerations.'

Comparing good scientific stuff with boring repetitive articles about minor problems as well as comparing accomplished poems with boring non-communicative stanza after stanza, it can be stated that the common denominator of quality, of goodness, is in both cases the notion of a little discovery, a discovery which is going to stay and attract our attenton also in the future, in other situations and in different contexts. And the longing to make the little discovery and prediction is, I feel, the primary motivation of both the scientific and poetic action. William Carlos Williams: 'Invent (if you can) discover or / nothing is clear — will surmount / the drumming in your head . . .'

So too the Czech modernist poet Vítězslav Nezval: 'And the aesthetic rule that once caused a radical overthrow in art may be at other times a burden for inspiration, a galley lead. Therefore the principal marker of art which provokes our interest is the novelty' (1930).

If the result is good, and this may happen at times, the great feeling is conveyed even to the reader of the scientific report. William Carlos Williams has remarked in a poem: 'We / have / microscopic anatomy / of the whale. This is / reassuring.' I don't think that this poem is so ironic. For Williams has written too: 'So much / depends / upon / a red wheel / barrow . . .' and this is taken seriously by everybody.

Or in an example from a recent scientific event: S. T. Peale, P. M. Cassen and R. T. Reynolds published in *Science* (2 March 1979) a paper indicating that Jupiter's gravity, tugging the near side of Jupiter's satellite Io harder than the far side, would cause the interior of Io to yield and create friction and heating, the accumulated heat being sufficient to melt the core, so that widespread volcanism can be expected. They said: 'Voyager images of Io may reveal evidence for a planetary structure dramatically different from any previously observed.' Three days thereafter Voyager I reached Jupiter and transmitted pictures of Io's yellow, orange and white surface shaped by recent volcanic activity and, later, clouds rising from a giant volcano. The human satisfaction one obtains from this episode equals the satisfaction from a great poem; the poetic quality is in the elegance of the prediction and in the coincidence of timing of the publication and the Voyager I success. No poetic qualities could be found in the paper itself.

On the contrary, an idea which appears extremely attractive in its human message, in its face value and in its wording happens to be very dangerous and misleading in the scientific context. A recent example occurs to me. Somebody investigated the reason for frequent miscarriages in an area where men used to drag heavily loaded ships by ropes. The author examined the miscarried fetuses and found that they were preponderantly of male sex, tended to turn away from the placenta and held the umbilical cords in their hands and over their shoulder, as if they were ropes. This is definitely a very poetic idea. Confronted by the valid genetic notions on the inheritance of adaptive qualities, the idea is a disaster and the observation may be rather an example of wishful thinking and jumping to conclusions than of a scientific hard or soft fact. Human approaches do not count in science. The moral and aesthetic values emerge at the very beginning and at the very end of the scientific activity, not in its mechanism.

What, then, is the difference or the likeness of the human experience in the very act of science-making and poetry-making? Are there common roots in the so-called creative impulse and are there common enjoyments in these two activities which we have described as basically different in the uses of words and handling of meanings?

Let us follow the single steps schematically:

1. Decision to act. In the lab, there is hardly ever the chance to start something new, to ask a purely personal, independent question. What one starts with is a heavy burden of accumu-

lated literature which is supposed to be known. The statement of the question is determined by the literature, by the hard facts and by the gaps. However, the question still may be personal, since it depends also on one's own interests, instincts for what may be important, the history of the work done (the profile of the lab) and the self-evaluation (what can I do with my skills, what can I afford with the given intellectual capacities and with the given tools?). After many twists and revisions, suddenly the point appears: this hasn't been done yet, this is techncally feasible, this is going to work, and this may lead to some yes or no answers. The emergence of the theme has a definite emotional quality and brings some sort of a recurrent enthusiasm, which one experiences any time one gets to the bench and to the work.

A sort of subacute or chronic inspiration, tension, hope and fear. Like a gastric ulcer, which you don't speak about.

Now the poem: I cannot give here, of course, a generally valid psychological pattern. I have to refer to my own experience and rely on the vivisection of my own writing. The statement or, better, feeling of the theme is primarily here; the confrontation with the work done by the subject and by the others is secondary. The theme appears to me as a general metaphor, as a shift from the obvious to the parareal. Its emergence implies the instincts for self-evaluation and personal style. What is strongly felt is again that . . . yes, this is going to work, this may work, if . . . this may lead to a poem. The emergence of the theme is at times the function of a definite emotional state which appears to be both the trigger and the driving and unifying force. At any rate, the emergence of the theme is connected with the feelings of elation, pain, relief, and with the same sort of acute enthusiasm which keeps one at work, even if it is not done at once.

Something like controlled heart insufficiency, which you freely advertise.

The basic difference between the emergence of the scientific theme and the poem theme is the notion and necessity of purification, definition and linearity in the former, and the notion of necessity of the openness, ramification-potential and multilevel interaction in the latter. The scientific theme implies as much light as possible, the poetic one as many shadows as possible. If they are not here, they must be created, opened, found in the course of the poem. The basic likeness of both activities is the agreeable experience of the self, of the interior functioning, or even well-functioning machine. If this sounds heretical for poetry, I would refer to William Carlos Williams: The poem is a machine made of words.

The agreeable experience may be better denoted as the realization of inner freedom, of the freedom of choice, of one of the very few moments of existential freedom. I tried to define this feeling, common to the finding of the way in the lab and to the finding of the way of the poem, in my piece, 'On the Origin of Legal Power':

> This time,
> when houses sit on eggs
> of the little painted Easter death
> and the symphony orchestra
> is dug in behind the bushes,
>
> when bassoons and trombones
> loom up on the road,
> asking for alms bigger than
> the live weight of the body,
>
> and he, listening to
> the inner unison we used to know by heart,

to the tempest-in-the-teapot,
to this in-spite-of-all-that,

does not recognize the big city
because of the little flame,
does realize the fatigue of the mountain mass
face to face with a falling stone

and
at least this time
when asked, replies,

Yes, I can.

And goes
the way of the flute.

2. Doing it. In the lab, doing it is so complicated that it can be described in the simplest terms. In one of the few poems where I could really render something from the laboratory experience, I said:

> You ask the secret.
> It has just one name:
> again . . .

'Doing it', working in the lab, requires a lot of self-restraint and discipline, of mastering momentary impulses for variations and deviations of the work, of tolerance for pitfalls and uncertainties, for the provisorial and not-yet-accomplished, for boring repetitions of the same step, for a pedantic order of actions and thoughts. It is at times a lonely, stubborn and defensive endeavour: there are always, as S. J. Lec says, some Eskimos around who would advise the inhabitants of the Congo what to do during a hot summer. To this end, let me quote my poem 'The Truth':

[141]

He left, infallible, the door itself
    was bruised as he
    hit the mark,

We two sat awhile
    the figures in the protocols
    staring at us like
    green huge-headed beetles
    out of the crevices of evening.

The books stretched
    their spines,
the balance weighed just for the fun of it
    and the glass beads in the necklace
    of the god of sleep whispered together
    in the scales.

'Have you ever been right?' one of us asked.
'I haven't.'

Then we counted on.
It was late
And outside the smoky town, frosty and purple
climbed to the stars.

Now, 'doing the poem' involves psychological mechanisms which I am tempted to describe in almost analogous terms. Metaphorically, I would say, it means to run the lab in the mind, with discipline, with the utmost sense of order and style, allowing for new incoming associations and notions only if they keep to the preconceived framework of possible consequences. William Carlos Williams went as far as . . . 'This combination of order with discovery, with exploration and revelation, the vigor of sensual stimulation, is of the essence of art.' The whole process is happening in one spot and in one time, or at least in one unique inner atmosphere which may occur at different times. It feels rather as if 'it is being done' or 'it is doing it' than 'I am doing it.'

The pitfalls and errors in lab work can be made good and eradicated by repetitions. The pitfalls and errors in the poem lead more frequently to wreckage and abandonment. However, both activities involve the basic risk of possible definitive losing, up to the moment when one suddenly discovers that it works, in spite of all that.

3. 'Finding it', the moment of success, or at least what one takes to be the proof of fulfilment, the experience of the little discovery, which is virtually identical when looking into the microscope and seeing the expected (or at times the unexpected but meaningful) and when looking at the nascent organism of the poem. The emotional, aesthetic and existential value is the same. It is one of the few real joys in life.

A strong feeling of reality. So strong that I've never dared describe it. Maybe also because I do not have enough personal experience with this moment. Neither in the lab. Nor in poetry.

But in any case, I feel compelled by all that I know to answer the above-stated question positively. Yes, there is a common root of so-called creativity; there is the same experience of fulfilment and inner reward. Therefore I could never quite understand people asking, How can you do both these things that are basically so different? They are technically different, technically at opposite poles of the application of language, but emanate from the same deep level of the human urge, and the application of all available forces.

So far, I've tried to describe science-making and poem-making as if one was alone with the theme, alone with the work, alone with the result. In reality, one is at almost all times deeply immersed in the collective process of life and survival, caring and worrying, winning and losing. There is no such thing as a 'scientist' and there is no such thing as a 'poet'. One can pretend it, one may play the role, but the essence of 'being it' is realized only in the rare moments described. I tried to elaborate on this in 'Conversation with a Poet':

You are a poet? Yes, I am.
How do you know?
　　　　I have written a poem.
When you wrote the poem, it meant you were a poet. But now?
　　　　I shall write another poem some day.
Then you may again be a poet. But how will you know that it really is a poem?
　　　　It will be just like the last one.

In that case it will certainly not be a poem. A poem exists only once – it cannot be the same again.
　　　　I mean it will be just as good.

But you cannot mean that. The goodness of a poem exists only once and does not depend on you but on circumstances.
　　　　I imagine the circumstances will be the same.

If that is your opinion, you never were a poet and never will be. Why, then, do you think you are a poet?
　　　　Well, I really don't know . . .
　　　　But who are you?

I can't be in other people's skin and I can't judge; but for myself, I would say that I have spent 95 per cent of my time and energy in fighting my way through the wild vegetation of circumstances, looking for the tiny spots, for the little clearing where I eventually could really work, write or do research, albeit the second happens to be my profession.

Why, then, should it make so much difference, being the poet and being the scientist, when 95 per cent of our time we are really secretaries, telephonists, passers-by, carpenters, plumbers, privileged and underprivileged citizens, waiting patrons, applicants, household maids, clerks, commuters, offenders, listeners, drivers, runners, patients, losers, subjects and shadows?

There is a tremendous amount of amateurism in everyday life and in professional life. The tension between the husks of unprofessional tasks and burdens and the kernels of professionalism is the most frequent tension in our experience. Our hard-centred scientific approach, as well as our soft-centred artistic approach, appears to be of little use in solving both the profane and the deepest troubles of our lives in moments of urgent need, alarm, crisis and desolation.

We pretend to live inside a world-fruit of our creativity and culture. But in fact our work happens to be a tiny, subtle, at times permeating, but most of the time confined domain in a world and in an age dominated by the giants of management and manipulation, by untamed autonomous superstructures which look down at us as if at an easily manageable microbial culture.

And this is the last aspect of reality where there is a total amalgamation of science and poetry: some sort of actual or potential hope in the world of autarchic actions. And this is exactly what we quoted from Oppenheimer: 'mutually exclusive ways of using our words . . . minds . . . souls . . . ways as different . . . as preparing to act and entering into retrospective search for the reasons of action . . .'

[145]

Let me conclude, therefore, with my 'Brief Reflection on the Test Tube':

You take
    a bit of fire, a bit of water,
    a bit of rabbit or tree,
    or any little piece of man,
    you mix it, shake well, cork it up,
    put it in a warm place, in darkness, in light, in frost,
    leave it alone for a while –
    though things don't leave you alone –
    and that's the whole point.

And then
    you have a look – and it grows,
    a little sea, a little volcano,
    a little tree, a little heart, a little brain,
    so small you don't hear it pleads
    to be let out,
    and that's the whole point, not to hear.

Then you go
    and record it, all the minuses or
    all the pluses, some with an exclamation-mark,
    all the zeros, or all the numbers, some with an
        exclamation-mark,
    and the point is that the test tube
    is an instrument for changing question-
        into exclamation-marks,

And the point is
    that for the moment you forget
    you yourselves are

In the test tube.